Pocket Reference of Diagnosis and Management for the Speech-Language Pathologist

Pocket Reference of Diagnosis and Management for the Speech-Language Pathologist

Patricia F. White, M.A., CCC-SLP
Speech Pathologist, Rehabilitation Services, Department of Speech Pathology, Methodist Hospital Central, Memphis, Tennessee

Butterworth–Heinemann

Boston   Oxford   Johannesburg   Melbourne   New Delhi   Singapore

Every effort has been made to ensure that the drug dosage schedules within this text are accurate and conform to standards accepted at time of publication. However, as treatment recommendations vary in the light of continuing research and clinical experience, the reader is advised to verify drug dosage schedules herein with information found on product information sheets. This is especially true in cases of new or infrequently used drugs.

∞ Recognizing the importance of preserving what has been written, Butterworth–Heinemann prints its books on acid-free paper whenever possible.

Library of Congress Cataloging-in-Publication Data
White, Patricia F., 1958–
    Pocket reference of diagnosis and management for the speech
    –language pathologist / Patricia F. White.
        p.   cm.
    Includes bibliographical references and index.
    ISBN 0-7506-9818-7
    1. Speech therapy—Handbooks, manuals, etc.   2. Speech disorders-
-Handbooks, manuals, etc.   3. Language disorders—Handbooks,
manuals, etc.   I. Title.
    [DNLM: 1. Speech Disorders—handbooks.   2. Language Disorders-
-handbooks.   WL 39 W587p 1996]
    RC423.W486   1996
    616.85'5—dc21
    DNLM/DLC
for Library of Congress   96-39070
                                                                            CIP

British Library Cataloguing-in-Publication Data
A catalogue record for this book is available from the British Library.

The publisher offers special discounts on bulk orders of this book.

For information, please contact:
Manager of Special Sales
Butterworth–Heinemann
313 Washington Street
Newton, MA 02158–1626   For information on all B-H medical publica-
Tel: 617-928-2500   tions available, contact our World Wide Web
Fax: 617-928-2620   home page at: http://www.bh.com/med

10 9 8 7 6 5 4 3 2

Printed in the United States of America

Contents

Preface

Having supervised many graduate students and clinical fellows in the field of speech-language pathology during the past 14 years, I became aware that our field lacked a source for immediate access to information to help diagnose and manage the diverse populations that our profession is now asked to serve. After fumbling for years with pages of information from short courses and tables copied from books secured to a clipboard, I thought it was finally time for someone to combine that information into a useable form.

This book was written with the intent of providing the clinician with a quick reference to pertinent information needed to diagnose and treat patients. It is not meant to replace textbooks, reference books, or a good educational background. In order to organize the contents in a convenient-sized handbook, not all the material can be covered in great detail.

This book was also written with the "traveling" clinician in mind: the clinician who sees patients bedside or in the home or the one who travels from facility to facility without the luxury of having an office close by with a library of reference materials. Not everyone will find all the information useful, but it is hoped the majority of the book will provide information you will need on a daily basis.

Some of the disorders covered in this book require the clinician to obtain special training before treating a patient. For example, assessing and treating infants in the neonatal intensive care unit, tracheoesophageal puncture fitting, and dysphagia assessment and treatment should be performed only by those having specific training in such areas.

I would like to thank the other professionals who were so generous with their ideas, comments, and knowledge during the writing of this book.

This book is dedicated to my friend and husband, Roger, and to my daughter, Amanda, both of whom are always a constant source of inspiration.

PFW

1

Aphasia and Related Disorders

Aphasia is a language disturbance that results from a disruption of the blood supply to the brain, as in a stroke, abnormal growth of the brain tissue (i.e., a tumor), or trauma to the brain caused by a head injury. The aphasic patient demonstrates difficulty in the production of spoken and written language, the comprehension of spoken and written language, or both. Not all patients with aphasia fit neatly into a particular category; some have generalized aphasias that overlap several types. This overlap can be attributed to multiple or extensive lesions or to lesions that have occurred in a brain already impaired by previous lesions or the aging process. These brain lesions may also result in other disorders, such as dementia, dysarthria, and apraxia, all of which can make a differential diagnosis difficult [1].

To understand aphasia, one must first have an understanding of how language is organized in the brain. Table 1.1 provides an outline of the lobes of the brain and their language functions. The major anatomical components of central language are listed in Table 1.2 and are shown in Figures 1.1 and 1.2.

TABLE 1.1. The lobes of the brain and their functions

Lobe	Function	Results of damage
Bilateral frontal lobe	Maturation Inhibits lower centers Complex interpretation Flexibility	Memory impairments Behavioral and personality changes Slower to react Difficulty learning new things Impaired judgment Poor strategic planning Impaired insight
Left or dominant frontal lobe	Motor programming Expressive language	Apraxia of speech Ideomotor apraxia Broca's aphasia Transcortical motor aphasia
Left or dominant parietal lobe	Left and right discrimination Map following Telling time Mathematics skills	Constructional apraxia Manually clumsy Poor ability to copy or draw letters Finger agnosia Difficulty understanding logical and spatial relationships Paraphasias Astereognosis Acalculia Written spelling errors exceed oral spelling errors Alexia with agraphia Body image impairments

Region	Functions	Disorders
Right or nondominant parietal lobe	Depth perception Colors and hues Recognizing forms by touch Spatial relations	Ideomotor apraxia Gerstmann's syndrome (may be due to a bilateral lesion) Right and left disorientation Ideational apraxia Hemispatial neglect Dressing apraxia Spatial and temporal disorientation Hemispatial neglect Disturbance of body schema Astereognosis Constructional apraxia Left neglect Flat affect Anosognosia
Left or dominant temporal lobe	Obtains, processes, and stores information Decodes sounds Interprets syntax and semantics Superior lobe for reading skills	Decreased auditory comprehension Auditory agnosia (usually due to a bilateral lesion) Decreased auditory memory Decreased reading comprehension Pure word deafness (usually a bilateral lesion) Wernicke's aphasia Anomic aphasia
Right or nondominant temporal lobe	Interprets environmental sounds Interprets emotional sounds (e.g., sarcasm, inflections)	Disturbance to the functions listed Pure word deafness (usually a bilateral lesion) Amusia

TABLE 1.1. (continued)

Lobe	Function	Results of damage
Left occipital lobe	Interprets nonverbal cues Visual analysis and synthesis	Visual field deficits Cortical blindness Hemianopsia Scanning impairments Visual agnosia (usually due to a bilateral lesion) Alexia without agraphia
Right occipital lobe	Ability to recognize one's own possessions Object and form recognition Recognition of familiar faces	Color agnosia Prosopagnosia (usually due to a bilateral lesion)

Source: AD Davis. A Survey of Adult Aphasia. Englewood Cliffs, NJ: Prentice-Hall, 1983; MS Burns, AS Halper, SI Mogil. Clinical Management of Right Hemisphere Dysfunction. Rockville, MD: Aspen, 1985; LL LaPointe. Aphasia and Related Neurologic Language Disorders. New York: Thieme, 1990; J Nolte. The Human Brain. St. Louis: Mosby, 1981; and RL Strub, FW Black. The Mental Status Examination in Neurology (3rd ed). Philadelphia: FA Davis, 1993.

TABLE 1.2. Major components of the central language mechanism model

Language areas	Function
Broca's area	Motor programming for articulation
Motor strip	Activates muscles for articulation
Arcuate fasciculus	Transmits linguistic information to anterior areas from posterior areas
Wernicke's area	Comprehension of oral language
Angular gyrus	Integrates visual, auditory, and tactile information Symbolic integration for reading
Supramarginal gyrus	Symbolic integration for writing
Corpus callosum	Transmits information between hemispheres
Subcortical areas	
Thalamus	Naming and memory mechanisms
Internal capsule, striatum, globus pallidus	Language and speech mechanisms

Source: Reprinted with permission from RJ Love, WG Webb. Neurology for the Speech-Language Pathologist (2nd ed). Boston: Butterworth–Heinemann, 1992;184.

An accurate identification of aphasia is the first step in delivering effective treatment. A catalog of aphasic symptoms can enhance the clinician's sensitivity to the variations in aphasic behavior. Table 1.3 provides the clinician with a quick reference to the cortical aphasia symptoms. One patient may exhibit only a few of these symptoms, whereas another patient may exhibit a different combination of symptoms. A patient's symptoms may also change during the recovery period. As recovery occurs, some of the characteristics may lessen or disappear as others emerge. An awareness of these possibilities assists the clinician in differentiating between types of aphasias, differentiating

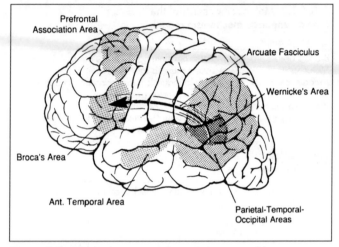

Figure 1.1. Primary language and association areas of the cortex. (Reprinted with permission from RJ Love, WG Webb. Neurology for the Speech-Language Pathologist [3rd ed]. Boston: Butterworth–Heinemann,1996;24.)

aphasic behavior from other disorders, and monitoring the stages of recovery. Aphasic symptoms also provide information about the etiology of the patient's disorder, which enables the clinician to plan treatment strategies that are the most appropriate for the individual's problem.

Aphasia syndromes can be broadly divided into two major categories based on the amount of verbal expression: nonfluent and fluent. The aphasias that are characterized by limited verbal expression are nonfluent aphasias and include Broca's aphasia, transcortical motor aphasia, and

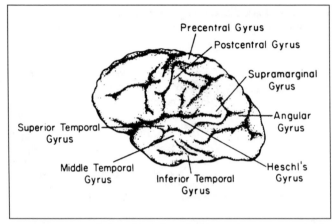

Figure 1.2. Lateral view of the left cerebral hemisphere. (Reprinted with permission from RJ Love, WG Webb. Neurology for the Speech-Language Pathologist [3rd ed]. Boston: Butterworth-Heinemann,1996;21.)

global aphasia. Fluent aphasias are characterized by greater verbal output (although it may be extremely impaired) and include Wernicke's aphasia, anomic aphasia, conduction aphasia, and transcortical sensory aphasia.

NONFLUENT APHASIAS

Broca's Aphasia

Lesion site: Lateral frontal lobe, prerolandic, suprasylvian region, extending into the adjacent subcortical periventricular white matter of the left or dominant hemisphere (see Figure 1.1) [2]

TABLE 1.3. Quick checklist of general cortical aphasia characteristics

| Characteristic | Type of aphasia | | |
	Broca's	Transcortical motor	Global
Conversational speech	Nonfluent	Nonfluent	Nonfluent
Auditory comprehension	Relatively normal	Good	Severely impaired
Repetition skills	Impaired	Good	Severely impaired
Word retrieval	Impaired	Impaired	Severely impaired
Reading comprehension	May be normal or impaired	Good	Severely impaired
Reading aloud	Impaired	Impaired	Severely impaired
Writing	Impaired	Impaired	Severely impaired
Hemiparesis	Yes	Yes	Yes, severe

Wernicke's	Anomic	Conduction	Transcortical sensory
Fluent	Fluent	Fluent	Fluent
Severely impaired	Relatively normal	Relatively normal	Severely impaired
Severely impaired	Good	Impaired	Good
Severely impaired	Impaired	Impaired	Impaired
Impaired	Relatively normal	Good	Impaired
Impaired	Relatively normal	Impaired	May be intact or impaired
Impaired	Relatively normal	Impaired	Impaired
No	No	No	Rare

Characteristics

- Telegraphic or agrammatic speech
- Restricted vocabulary and grammar
- Awkward articulation (distortions)
- Written language errors that reflect spoken language errors
- Speech requires effort
- Poor syntax
- Absence of prepositions, pronouns, adjectives, or adverbs
- Short bursts of speech
- Shows awareness of errors
- Relatively normal auditory comprehension
- Difficulty with repetition and naming tasks
- Repetition and reading aloud as impaired as conversational speech

Other Symptomatology

- Right hemiplegia
- Aphasia usually accompanied by verbal apraxia

*Transcortical Motor Aphasia**

Lesion site: Anterior and superior to Broca's area, but not as extensive as the lesion causing Broca's aphasia; anterior

---

*Transcortical motor aphasia may be confused with Broca's aphasia because both are characterized by poor expressive language skills and good comprehension. To differentiate between the two, note that verbal production during repetition tasks in transcortical motor aphasia is far better than that found in Broca's aphasia.

border zone lesion between the territories of the anterior and middle cerebral arteries

Characteristics

- Absence of spontaneous speech and inability to initiate speech
- Echolalic speech
- Good repetition skills
- Poor word-retrieval skills in naming tasks
- Relatively normal auditory comprehension
- Poor oral reading
- Relatively normal reading comprehension
- Correct articulation
- Poor writing skills

Other Symptomatology

- Urinary incontinence
- Rigidity of the upper extremity
- Hemiparesis involving the leg more than the arm
- Initial mutism that quickly evolves into transcortical motor aphasia
- Bilateral motor apraxia
- Slowness of movement

Global Aphasia

Lesion site: Broca's and Wernicke's areas; usually involves the middle cerebral artery (see Figure 1.1)

Characteristics

- Severely impaired auditory comprehension
- Severe impairment in understanding and imitating gross motor movements
- Conversational speech absent or reduced to a few stereotyped words or sounds
- Repetition skills at the same level as conversational speech
- Severe agraphia, alexia, and acalculia

Other Symptomatology

- Severe hemiparesis
- Urinary incontinence
- Usually accompanied by an oral-verbal apraxia
- Dysarthria possible

FLUENT APHASIAS

Wernicke's Aphasia

Lesion sites: Angular and supramarginal gyri of the parietal lobe and on the posterior portion of the superior temporal gyrus in the left or dominant hemisphere (see Figures 1.1 and 1.2)

Characteristics

- Severely impaired auditory comprehension
- Tendency for excessive speech; lack of conversational turn-taking

- Auditory agnosia
- Short auditory memory
- Verbal language that contains jargon
- Paraphasias
- Auditory comprehension more impaired than speech output
- Fluent articulation and speech
- Poor word-retrieval skills in naming tasks
- Poor oral reading and reading comprehension skills
- Poor writing skills
- Unaware of mistakes
- Poor repetition skills

Other Symptomatology

- Absence of hemiparesis
- Initially euphoric, but may become paranoid later
- Bizarre speech and absence of other apparent neurologic symptoms (Patient may initially be misdiagnosed as psychotic due to these symptoms.)

Transcortical Sensory Aphasia

Lesion site: Posterior parieto-temporal area (border zone of Wernicke's area) (see Figure 1.1)

Characteristics

- Remarkable repetition ability
- Inability to find words
- Initiates little speech

- Echolalic
- Good automatic speech skills
- Severely impaired auditory comprehension
- Verbal language that contains jargon
- Paraphasias
- Poor word-retrieval skills in naming tasks
- Poor reading comprehension skills
- Oral reading intact, masking poor reading comprehension
- Poor writing skills

Other Symptomatology

- Alexia
- Constructional apraxia
- Ideational apraxia
- Hemiparesis rarely noted

Anomic Aphasia

Lesion sites: Second temporal gyrus, angular gyrus (see Figure 1.2)

Characteristics

- Poor word-retrieval skills in naming tasks
- No paraphasias
- Good repetition skills
- Relatively normal auditory comprehension
- Uses circumlocutions well

Conduction Aphasia

Lesion sites: Arcuate fasciculus and supramarginal gyrus, or damage to the insula, contiguous auditory cortex, and underlying white matter (see Figures 1.1 and 1.2) [3]

Characteristics

- Fluent yet halting speech with word-finding pauses
- Repetition skills impaired
- Good auditory comprehension skills
- Literal and phonemic paraphasias
- Shows awareness of errors
- Articulation worsens with repetition
- Struggles to untangle words
- Oral reading impaired
- Reading comprehension intact
- Writing skills marked by errors in spelling, word choice, and syntax

SUBCORTICAL APHASIA [2]

Anterior Capsular/Putaminal Aphasia

Lesion site: Anterior portion of the internal capsule

Characteristics

- Has features of both transcortical motor and Broca's aphasias
- Good auditory comprehension

- Short phrase length
- Relatively good repetition skills
- Hemiplegia
- Poor verbal and nonverbal agility

Posterior Capsular/Putaminal Aphasia

Lesion site: Posterior portion of the internal capsule

Characteristics

- Has features of both Broca's and Wernicke's aphasias
- Poor repetition skills
- Hemiplegia
- Poor auditory comprehension
- Good articulatory agility but poor nonverbal agility

Global Capsular/Putaminal Aphasia

Lesion sites: Small anterior and posterior capsular/putaminal lesion

Characteristics

- Global-like syndrome
- Poor auditory comprehension
- Little or no verbal output

Thalamic Aphasia

Lesion site: Thalamus

Characteristics

- Has features of both transcortical motor and transcortical sensory aphasias
- Relatively good repetition skills
- Variable articulatory agility
- Conversational speech inertia
- Variable auditory comprehension
- Semantic paraphasias
- Hemiplegia

BLOOD SUPPLY TO THE CORTEX

A cerebrovascular accident (CVA) is a disruption of the blood flow to the brain. A CVA can occur due to a thrombosis, embolism, or hemorrhage.

Because most cases of aphasia are caused by CVAs, it is essential to understand the structure of the blood flow to the brain. Different patterns of symptoms and different expectations for recovery are related to the location of the damage in the arterial system.

Three cerebral arteries cover the surface of each hemisphere of the brain. The anterior cerebral artery supplies the medial surface of the cortex. The middle cerebral artery (MCA) branches to most of the lateral cortex. The posterior cerebral artery covers the medial surface of the occipital lobe and the base of the temporal lobe. The cerebral arteries are shown in Figure 1.3.

The three cerebral arteries originate from an anastomotic circle of arteries at the base of the brain. This sys-

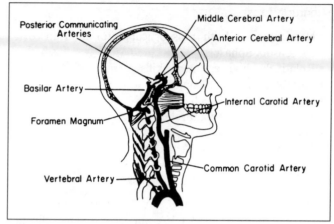

Figure 1.3. Cerebral arteries. (Redrawn and reproduced with permission from R Snell. Clinical Neuroanatomy for Medical Students. Boston: Little, Brown, 1980.)

tem is called the circle of Willis and is formed by the anterior communicating artery, the two anterior cerebral arteries, the two internal carotid arteries, the two posterior communicating arteries, the two posterior cerebral arteries, and the basilar artery (Figure 1.4). The circle of Willis is supplied by both sides of arteries in the neck, the two internal carotid arteries, and the two vertebral arteries. Each internal artery connects to its respective MCA. Therefore, the internal carotid supplies the lateral and anterior portions of the brain through its direct connec-

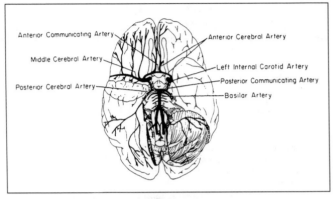

Figure 1.4. Circle of Willis. (Redrawn and reproduced with permission from R Snell. Clinical Neuroanatomy for Medical Students. Boston: Little, Brown, 1980.)

tion with the MCA and its indirect connection with the anterior cerebral artery. The vertebral arteries are joined, becoming the basilar artery, which supplies blood to the posterior circle of Willis.

The circle of Willis acts as a protective mechanism that allows for collateral circulation to the brain. Collateral circulation allows the brain to compensate for reduced blood flow should an artery become occluded. It also allows blood to flow across the midline of the brain if an artery on one side becomes occluded. The neurologic

TABLE 1.4. Neurologic deficits associated with cerebral artery damage

When a CVA occurs in the **middle cerebral artery**, the patient may experience the following:

Aphasia

Alexia

Agraphia

Visual field deficits

Contralateral hemiparesis (more severe in the face and arm than in the leg)

Altered level of consciousness

Contralateral sensory deficit

When a CVA occurs in the **internal carotid artery**, the patient may experience the following:

Headaches

Weakness, paralysis, numbness, sensory changes, and visual deficits (e.g., blurring on the affected side)

Altered level of consciousness

Aphasia

Ptosis

When a CVA occurs in the **anterior cerebral artery**, the patient may experience the following:

Confusion

Weakness and numbness on the affected side

Paralysis of the contralateral foot and leg

Footdrop

Incontinence

Loss of coordination

Impaired sensory functions

Personality changes

When a CVA occurs in the **vertebral or basilar artery**, the patient may experience the following:

Numbness around the lips and mouth

Dizziness

Weakness on the affected side

Visual deficits (i.e., color blindness, lack of depth perception, and diplopia)

Poor coordination

Dysphagia
Dysarthria
Amnesia
Ataxia
Coma or confusion
Impaired gag reflex
Headache
When a CVA occurs in the **posterior cerebral artery**, the patient may
experience the following:
Visual field deficits
Sensory impairment
Alexia
Coma
Cortical blindness from ischemia in the occipital area
"Locked in" syndrome, during which the patient is in a state of complete
paralysis, except for some form of voluntary eye movement
Achromatopsia
Alexia without agraphia
Environmental agnosia

CVA = cerebrovascular accident.
Source: Adapted from S Loeb (ed). Nursing TimeSavers: Neurologic Disorders. Springhouse, PA: Springhouse, 1994;186.

deficits associated with damage to the various cerebral
arteries are provided in Table 1.4.

APHASIA TERMINOLOGY AND OTHER
RELATED DISORDERS OF APHASIA

The following disorders are considered to be related to
aphasia because they are caused by damage to the nervous
system and may interfere with communication. It is important to identify and differentiate these disorders because
they may either accompany aphasia or be confused with

aphasia. Such disorders require different therapy approaches for rehabilitation.

Acalculia — The patient experiences a disturbance in mathematics ability, resulting in the loss of understanding of the significance of numbers or an inability to perform mathematics functions. The ability to tell time and make change may also be disturbed. This disorder is distinct from the inability to read or write numbers.

Achromatopsia — Central achromatopsia is the loss of color vision due to a brain lesion. The achromatopsia is limited to the hemifield contralateral to the lesion that damages the inferomedial occipital region anterior to the visual cortex. Infarction in the distribution of the posterior cerebral artery is the most common cause of central achromatopsia, but the syndrome can also be caused by brain tumors and other focal lesions involving the ventromedial occipital cortex [4].

Agrammatism — The patient experiences a disturbance in the ability to order words in their correct sequence and has difficulty with grammar and syntax.

Agraphia — The patient suffers from a disorder of writing caused by lesions in the dominant parietal lobe, frontal language area, and (rarely) the anterior corpus callosum. Most patients with aphasia demonstrate some degree of agraphia.

Alexia — A previously literate patient experiences a disturbance in the ability to understand the meaning of written words and sentences. *See* Alexia without agraphia.

Alexia with agraphia — The patient is unable to read or write. Damage is in the inferior parietal lobule (angular gyrus and environs) [3].

Alexia without agraphia — The patient is able to understand words spelled aloud and write meaningful sentences but is unable to read his or her writing. Pure alexia without agraphia is caused by either a left posterior cerebral artery occlusion in a right-handed patient, which damages a portion of the posterior corpus callosum and the left occipital lobe, or a bilateral lesion involving the inferior temporal occipital junction and subjacent white matter. Either type of damage results in the disconnection of the inferior parietal lobule from all visual input [3]. Alexia without agraphia is also known as pure alexia and pure word blindness.

Alzheimer's disease — This disease is one of the most common forms of dementia. It is a type of mental deterioration characterized by both disorientation and impaired memory, judgment, and intellect. Initial symptoms are apathy, memory difficulties, constructional impairment, acalculia, and problems with abstract reasoning. Later symptoms include anomia, apraxia, agnosia, geographic disorientation, and significant deficits in judgment (see Chapter 5).

Amusia — The patient experiences the total or partial inability to produce or to comprehend musical sounds.

Anarthria — The patient loses of the ability to speak. Anarthria can result from a brain lesion or damage to the peripheral nerves that innervate the articulatory muscles.

Anosognosia — The patient denies illness. Anosognosia can vary from an underestimation of deficits to a complete denial of any deficit. It usually occurs with right parietal lesions, and involves denial of the contralateral hemiparesis, hemisensory loss, or visual field deficit.

Anterograde amnesia — The patient is unable to learn new material. Anterograde amnesia is a post-traumatic disorder.

Apraxia — The patient is unable to sequence voluntary motor movements. Apraxia is not due to disturbances of strength, coordination, sensation, or a lack of comprehension or attention (see Chapter 3).

Astereognosis — The patient is unable to recognize an object using the sense of touch. Astereognosis is usually due to a lesion in the anterior portion of the parietal lobe (involving the postcentral gyrus) opposite the astereognostic hand. In rare cases, the lesion may be in the anterior corpus callosum [3]. Also known as tactile agnosia.

Auditory agnosia — The patient has an impaired ability to comprehend language, nonlanguage sounds (environmental sounds), or both.

Autotopagnosia — The patient is unable to recognize any part of his or her body. Autotopagnosia is caused by a lesion of the dominant hemisphere. It is also known as somatotopagnosis.

Capgras' syndrome — A syndrome that is characterized by the delusional belief that a person or persons have been substituted by an impostor. It is caused by right hemisphere damage, post-traumatic encephalopathy, epilepsy, cerebrovascular disease, and a variety of other neurologic disorders [4].

Color agnosia — The patient is unable to recognize colors. The patient fails to point to colors on command, to name colors, and to name the color of color-specific objects such as a banana or carrot. Color discrimination is preserved. This disorder may be a specific color-naming disturbance caused by a lesion that disconnects visual input from the language area. (This type is associated with the syndrome alexia with agraphia.) A second type is an impairment of color perception caused by bilateral inferior temporo-occipital lesions. Most patients with the second type also have a prosopagnosia [3].

Creutzfeldt-Jakob disease — This disease is a form of subacute spongiform encephalopathy caused by a slow virus. The encephalopathy progresses rapidly to coma and death. The disease is characterized by dementia, myoclonus, ataxia, and other neurologic disturbances.

Dysarthria — A motor speech disorder that is characterized by weakness of the muscles that control articulation, respiration, resonation, prosody, and phonation (see Chapter 3).

Environmental agnosia — The patient experiences a loss of environmental familiarity and the inability to become topographically oriented even in familiar surroundings. Intellect and memory are intact. The lesion necessary to produce environmental agnosia is an inferomedial temporo-occipital lesion in the right hemisphere. It is usually due to right posterior cerebral artery infarctions, but the syndrome has occurred with other etiologies [4].

Finger agnosia — The patient is unable to recognize, name, and point to his or her or other's individual fingers. It may result from diffuse or focal brain disease seen in association with aphasia, apraxia, right-left disorientation, or general dementia. It is usually due to lesions in the parietal-occipital lobes of the dominant hemisphere.

Gerstmann's syndrome — This neurologic syndrome consists of four major components: finger agnosia, right-left disorientation, dysgraphia, and dyscalculia. It is caused by lesions to the dominant parietal lobe or to bilateral parietal lobes.

Hemiacalculia — The patient detects only half of a series of numbers in the calculation process. This deficit is usually found in patients suffering from right hemisphere damage [4].

Hemialexia — The patient reads only half of a word or sentence—for example, he or she may read "mailman" as "man." This deficit is usually found in patients suffering from right hemisphere damage [4].

Hemianopsia — The patient experiences loss of vision in one-half of the visual field of one or both eyes. It is also known as hemianopia.

Hemispatial neglect — The patient fails to detect, report, or orient to stimuli in one hemiuniverse. The neglect is contralateral to the lesion. It can result from either right or left hemisphere parietal, frontal, or subcortical lesions. The effects of this disorder are most severe with parietal lesions and most persistent with right-hemisphere damage. A hemispatial neglect is independent of the existence of a visual field deficit.

Jargon — Lengthy, fluently articulated utterance that makes little or no sense to the listener. It contains verbal paraphasias and neologisms and is commonly seen in global aphasia and Wernicke's aphasia.

Korsakoff's syndrome — This syndrome is a degenerative brain disease that results from a thiamine deficit seen in alcoholism or severe malnutrition and is characterized by severe recent memory deficits.

Nonverbal amnesia — The patient is unable to recall nonverbal visual material. This syndrome can result from right hemisphere lesions. Right temporal lobectomy results in impairment of retention of complex visual patterns and faces. Right thalamic lesions can also disrupt nonverbal memory [4].

Object agnosia — The patient is unable to recognize objects and their use. It results in the patient's inability to perform everyday activities such as making a bed or cooking a meal. This disorder is usually associated with widespread intellectual deterioration. It is also known as ideational apraxia (see Chapter 3).

Organic brain syndrome — This syndrome is characterized by a constellation of behavioral or psychological signs and symptoms caused by transient or permanent brain dysfunction. Alzheimer's disease is the most prevalent cause.

Pick's disease — This disease is a dementing illness resulting from atrophy of the frontal and temporal lobes of the brain. Motor speech impairments are often the first symptoms.

Prosopagnosia — The patient is unable to recognize previously known people, famous people, and people he or she has just met. The patient should be able to recognize the person on hearing the person's voice. The lesion is usually in the occipitotemporal areas bilaterally. One of the lesions is usually in the right inferior temporo-occipital region.

Pure word deafness — The patient experiences a total lack of speech comprehension without deficits in expressive language, agraphia, or alexia. The patient's hearing is intact, and he or she recognizes environmental sounds. The lesion is located in the posterior language area in the temporal lobe and is usually bilateral.

Pure word blindness — *See* Alexia without agraphia.

Reduplicative paramnesia — The patient experiences a disorder of spatial orientation. The patient insists that a current unfamiliar environment is located closer to a place that is more important and familiar (e.g., the patient feels the hospital room is right outside his or her house). Patients usually have impaired spatial perception, poor visual memory, and an inability to recognize inappropriate responses. The syndrome is usually caused by a combination of either right parietal and bilateral frontal injuries, or right parietal damage and an acute confusional state. Reduplicative paramnesia is also known as environmental reduplication [4].

Retrograde amnesia — The patient is unable to remember events that occurred before the brain injury that caused the amnesia.

Right hemisphere syndrome — This syndrome is a cluster of deficits usually seen in patients who have right hemisphere brain damage. It is characterized by impulsivity, left neglect, disorientation of time and place, denial of deficits, decreased judgment and reasoning, flat affect, deficits in visuospatial perception, and altered body concepts.

Somatotopagnosis — The inability to identify any part of the body, whether one's own or another's body. Somatotopagnosis is also known as autotopagnosia and somatagnosia [5].

Tactile agnosia — *See* Astereognosis

Unilateral hemianopsia — The loss of sight in one-half of the visual field of only one eye due to a lesion in the visual cortex.

Visual agnosia — This is a rare disorder that impairs the recognition of objects or pictures of objects presented visually. It is not due to any visual acuity problem. The patient is mentally clear and aphasia is absent. Patients can readily identify the object once it is handed to them through kinesthetic cues. Damage is to the visual association cortex bilaterally or to a bilateral lesion involving the inferior temporal occipital junction and subjacent white matter. The damage can also be caused by an infarct that destroys the left occipital lobe and the posterior corpus callosum. This disorder is usually seen in patients who are also alexic [3].

Visual object agnosia — The patient can see the object but cannot name it, demonstrate its function, or remember having seen it before. The patient can use the name in conversation and can retrieve the name when stimulated through other modalities such as touching the object.

PROGNOSTIC INDICATORS

In some respects, making prognostic predictions is a guessing game because of the variations between patients. The amount and rate of recovery can differ dramatically between patients. The major recovery indicators are the etiology, the site of the lesion, the size of the lesion, the type of aphasia, and the initial severity of the aphasia.

ETIOLOGY. A traumatic injury, especially closed head injuries, can result in better and more rapid recovery than an ischemic CVA.

SITE. Damage to marginal areas produces a more complete and a more rapid rate of recovery than damage to primary language areas. A CVA in the middle cerebral artery or trauma to the primary language areas generally produces permanent aphasia.

SIZE AND TYPE. Large infarcts (e.g., those found in global aphasia) generally have poor outcomes because there is too much damage for recovery to occur.

SEVERITY. The initial severity of the deficit is related to the size and location of the brain lesion. Severity of auditory comprehension deficit may be the most useful predictor of overall outcome [1].

There are other factors that interact with the ones mentioned above, thus influencing a patient's recovery. A patient with moderate deficits who is severely depressed may have a less favorable outcome than a patient with moderate deficits who is highly motivated, outgoing, and has a good family support system. Each case should be evaluated in light of all of the issues.

Negative Prognostic Indicators

- Severe initial impairments
- Severe auditory comprehension deficits
- Severe oral apraxia one month after stroke
- Total inability to communicate through oral speech
- Severe dysarthria
- Severe disturbance in verbal repeating tasks
- Depression
- Poor motivation
- Poor family support
- Low premorbid education level
- Other medical complications
- History of previous stroke

Favorable Prognostic Indicators

- Expressing ideas well

- Good ability to self-correct
- Good oral spelling
- Large amounts of spontaneous recovery
- Young patient
- High degrees of initial auditory comprehension
- High motivation
- Good family support
- Good premorbid education level

REFERENCES

1. Davis AD. A Survey of Adult Aphasia. Englewood Cliffs, NJ: Prentice-Hall, 1983;1,32,209.
2. Estabrooks NH, Albert ML. Manual of Aphasia Therapy. Austin, TX: PRO-ED, 1991;19.
3. Strub RL, Black FW. The Mental Status Examination in Neurology (3rd ed). Philadelphia: FA Davis, 1993;48,L45.
4. Burns MS, Halper AS, Mogil SI. Clinical Management of Right Hemisphere Dysfunction. Rockville, MD: Aspen, 1985;9.
5. Hensyl WR, Felscher H, Cady B (eds). Stedman's Medical Dictionary (25th ed). Baltimore: Williams & Wilkins, 1990;1435.

SUGGESTED READING

LaPointe LL. Aphasia and Related Neurologic Language Disorders. New York: Thieme, 1990.

Love RJ, Webb WG. Neurology for the Speech-Language Pathologist (3rd ed). Boston: Butterworth-Heinemann, 1996.

Nolte J. The Human Brain. St. Louis: Mosby, 1981.

Snell R. Clinical Neuroanatomy for Medical Students. Boston: Little, Brown, 1980.

2

Brain Tumors

BRAIN TUMOR TYPES AND GRADES

The cause of primary brain tumors is still unknown. The peak incidences occur in early childhood and between the ages of 50 and 80 [1]. Along with stroke and trauma, brain tumor is a principal cause of aphasia. As benign brain tumors grow, they apply pressure to the adjacent brain tissue. Malignant tumors not only apply pressure, but also invade and destroy surrounding tissue. Tumors within the brain may infiltrate widely before destroying a specific location of brain tissue. Early symptoms of these neoplasms usually are very general reductions of function. Seizures, blurred vision, headaches, vomiting, and aphasia may be some of the first symptoms to emerge. Aphasic symptoms will differ depending on the type of tumor, its location, and its rate of growth.

Brain tumors may be classified as *primary* or *secondary* and as *malignant* or *benign*. They may also be classified by location, cellular origin, or histologic features. If malignant tumors are not discovered early and removed, prognosis is poor. Whether a tumor is benign or malignant, it can cause tissue destruction, distortion, and displacement. It can also compress blood vessels, obstruct the flow of cerebrospinal fluid, and increase intracranial pressure. These events can result in focal neurologic deficits, cerebral edema, tissue hypoxia, and even brain herniation [1, 2].

Primary tumors originate in the brain. Secondary brain tumors are caused by malignant cells from other cancerous sites in the body that metastasize to the brain. The most common origins for secondary tumors are the lungs, breasts, gastrointestinal tract, and kidneys [1].

Tumors classified by location include supratentorial tumors, which are located within the cerebral hemispheres, and infratentorial tumors, which are found within the brain stem and cerebellum. Tumors classified by cellular origin include glioblastomas, which arise from the glial cells; meningiomas, which arise from the meningeal layers that cover the brain; and neurofibromas, which arise from the nerve sheath surrounding the nerve fibers.

Grades

I	Well differentiated
II	Moderately differentiated
III and IV	Grossly undifferentiated

Types of Brain Tumors and Their Characteristics

Gliomas
  Astrocytomas
    Slow-growing glioma
    Seizures may be the initial symptom
    Usually occur in the frontal, temporal, or parietal
      lobes
    Prognosis: Life expectancy of 6–7 years after
      surgery
  Astrocytomas grades III and IV (also called glioblas-
    toma multiforme)
    Infiltrative tumor
    Frequently in the white matter of the anterior or
      frontal part of cerebral hemispheres
    Malignant
    Rapid-growing mass
    Likely to invade both sides of the brain through
      connecting pathways
    Peak incidence at 45–55 years of age
    Most common primary tumor in adults
    Prognosis: Life expectancy of usually 12–18 months
      after surgery
  Ependymomas
    Occur in the ventricles (particularly the fourth
      ventricle)
    May grow into the cerebral hemisphere

       Prognosis: Life expectancy of 1 month after surgery
          if tumor is malignant, 7–8 years if it is benign
    Oligodendrogliomas
       Slow-growing
       Usually occur in frontal and temporal lobes
       Seizures typically the first symptom
       Prognosis: Life expectancy after surgery of 5 years
          or more
Cranial and spinal nerve and root tumors
    Acoustic neuromas
       Also called schwannoma or neurofibroma
       Occur in cranial nerve VIII, cerebellopontine angle
       Benign, slow-growing
       Large tumors may compress cranial nerves V, VII,
          IX, X
       Prognosis: usually good, excellent if the tumor is
          small and surgically accessible
Neural cell tumors
    Medulloblastomas
       Most often in cerebellar vermis
       Vision disturbances usually the first symptom
       Prognosis: Life expectancy is 5 years after surgery.
Mesodermal tissue tumors
    Meningiomas
       Second most common primary brain tumor in adults
       Arises from meningeal covering of the brain
       Peak incidence at 30–40 years of age
       Complete surgical removal possible
       Firm, slow-growing, encapsulated tumor

Prognosis: excellent, especially with complete
removal
Pituitary tumors
Pituitary adenomas
Most common in anterior lobe of pituitary gland
Usually benign, slow-growing
May cause visual disorders, headaches, and various
endocrine disorders
Prognosis: very good
Blood vessel tumors
Angiomas
Arise from congenitally malformed arteriovenous
connections
Occur primarily in the posterior cerebral hemi-
spheres
Slow-growing
May cause seizures, cerebral bleeding, and
increased intracranial pressure
Prognosis: good
Hemangioblastomas
Usually occur in cerebellum as a single or multiple
lesion
Occur less frequently in the medulla or cerebral
hemispheres
Vascular, slow-growing
Prognosis: excellent, usually curable
Congenital tumors
Craniopharyngiomas
More common in children

Located in or near the sella pituitary
Slow-growing, solid, or cystic tumors
Endocrine dysfunction common
Congenital
Prognosis: excellent if the tumor is removed [1]

Brain Tumor Sites and Associated Language and Sensory Deficits

Frontal lobe (see Table 1.1)
Parietal lobe (see Table 1.1)
Temporal lobe (see Table 1.1)
Occipital lobe (see Table 1.1)
Pituitary
   Visual field deficits
Pons
   Loss of ipsilateral facial or forehead sensation
   Loss of corneal reflex
Cranial nerves I, VI, VII, VIII, IX, X, XI, XII (see Table 4.1 for nerve deficits associated with brain tumors and other lesions)
Cerebellum
   Disturbed gait
   Impaired balance
   Loss of coordination
Midbrain
   Diplopia
   Ipsilateral inability to gaze up, down, or inward [1]

REFERENCES

1. Loeb S (ed). Nursing TimeSavers: Neurologic Disorders. Springhouse, PA: Springhouse, 1994;253.
2. Davis AD. A Survey of Adult Aphasia. Englewood Cliffs, NJ: Prentice-Hall, 1983.

SUGGESTED READING

Estabrooks NH, Albert ML. Manual of Aphasia Therapy. Austin, TX: PRO-ED, 1991;38.

REFERENCES

SUGGESTED READING

3

Motor Speech Disorders

DYSARTHRIA SYNDROMES AND THEIR CHARACTERISTICS

Dysarthria is a specific disorder of speech in which the muscles controlling articulation, respiration, phonation, prosody, and resonation are affected, while basic language remains intact. Dysarthrias can be caused by congenital injuries and anomalies, as well as a variety of acquired conditions (e.g., infections, toxic processes, space-occupying neoplasms, demyelinating diseases, neuromuscular diseases, trauma, and multiple varieties of cerebrovascular disturbances). Damage can be located in cortical areas, the cerebellum, the brain stem, or in the peripheral nervous system, which comprises the cranial and spinal nerves and their associated ganglia. The type of dysarthria caused by neurologic damage is determined by the site and extent of the lesion and when the insult occurs in the development of the patient [1].

Ataxic Dysarthria

Lesion site: Cerebellum
Causes: Stroke, cerebellar tumor, traumatic brain injury, ataxic cerebral palsy, Friedreich's ataxia, infection, and toxic effects of alcohol and other chemicals [1]

Characteristics

- Imprecise consonants
- Speech errors of timing
- Equal stress given to each syllable
- Overshooting and undershooting of articulators
- Voice quality is usually normal but can be harsh
- Monopitch, monoloudness
- Sudden bursts of loudness
- Coarse voice tremor
- Irregular articulation breakdowns
- Loss of muscle coordination, balance, and equilibrium
- Tremors during voluntary movement (intention tremors)

Flaccid Dysarthria

Lesion site: Lower motor neurons
Causes: Stroke and other cardiovascular diseases, myasthenia gravis, multiple sclerosis, muscular dystrophy, myopathies, lesions or tumors of the vagus nerve, trauma, Guillain-Barré syndrome, Möbius' syndrome, bulbar facial palsy and other palsies, tuberculosis, diphtheria, tetany, poliomyelitis and other viral infections, endotracheal intubation, bronchoscopy, granuloma [1–3]

Characteristics

- Breathy voice quality
- Weak vocal intensity
- Hypernasality
- Nasal emission
- Hypoactive gag reflex
- Weakened muscles of articulation
- Imprecise consonant formation
- Slow rate of speech

Hyperkinetic Dysarthria

Lesion site: Extrapyramidal system (basal ganglia)
Causes: Sydenham's chorea, Huntington's chorea, dystonia, organic voice tremor, palatopharyngeolaryngeal myoclonus, Gilles de la Tourette's syndrome, infection, ballism, athetosis, stroke, tumor, dystonia, prolonged use of psychotropic and antiparkinsonian drugs, dyskinesia [1–3]

Characteristics

- Quick, jerky, irregular, unpredictable movements
- Abnormal muscle tone (ranges from hypotonic to hypertonic)
- Inappropriate interruptions of phonation (voice arrests)
- Irregular pitch fluctuations
- Excess loudness variations
- Strained, strangled, or harsh voice quality
- Monopitch, monoloudness

- Imprecise consonants, distorted vowels
- Irregular articulation breakdowns
- Prolonged intervals
- Variable rate of speech

Hypokinetic Dysarthria

Lesion site: Extrapyramidal system (basal ganglia)
Causes: Parkinson's disease, drug side effects (e.g., chlorpromazine, fluphenazine) [1]

Characteristics

- Monopitch, monoloudness
- Reduced loudness
- Reduced stress
- Imprecise consonants
- Short rushes of speech (in patients with Parkinson's disease)
- Harsh, breathy voice quality
- Inappropriate silences
- Mask-like face (in patients with Parkinson's disease)
- Vocal tremor

Mixed (Spastic-Ataxic-Hypokinetic) Dysarthria

Lesion sites: Upper motor neuron, cerebellar, extrapyramidal
Causes: Wilson's disease [1]

Characteristics

- Monopitch, monoloudness

- Imprecise consonants
- Reduced stress
- Excess and equal stress
- Slow rate of speech
- Low-pitched voice
- Irregular articulation breakdowns

Mixed (Spastic-Flaccid) Dysarthria

Lesion sites: Vagus nerve, pyramidal tract
Causes: Amyotrophic lateral sclerosis, trauma, stroke [1]

Characteristics

- Harsh, strained, strangled voice quality
- Breathiness
- Short phrases
- Low-pitched voice
- Wet vocal quality
- Imprecise consonants and distorted vowels
- Hypernasality
- Audible inhalation, may have inhalation stridor
- Excess and equal stress
- Rapid tremor on vowel prolongation
- Reduced loudness
- Slow rate of speech
- Prolonged intervals
- Monopitch, monoloudness
- Inappropriate laughter or crying
- Tongue fasciculations

Spastic Dysarthria

Lesion site: Upper motor neuron
Causes: Pseudobulbar palsy, stroke, tumor, poliomyelitis, encephalitis and other infections, traumatic brain injury, multiple sclerosis, spastic cerebral palsy [1–3]

Characteristics

- Harsh, strained, strangled voice quality
- Abnormally low pitch
- Monopitch, monoloudness
- Reduced loudness
- Poor prosody
- Hypernasality
- Imprecise consonant formation
- Slow rate of speech
- Inappropriate laughing or crying

Variable (Spastic-Ataxic-Flaccid) Dysarthria

Lesion sites (variable): Upper motor neuron, cerebellum, lower motor neuron
Causes: Multiple sclerosis [1]

Characteristics

- Slow rate of speech
- Harsh voice quality
- Irregular articulation breakdowns

APRAXIA SYNDROMES AND THEIR CHARACTERISTICS

Apraxia is the inability to perform volitional motor movements in the presence of normal comprehension, muscle strength, sensation, attention, and coordination. Apraxia results from a lesion that disconnects Broca's area from the motor association area responsible for organizing intentional actions [3]. "Pure" apraxias are rarely seen. Many patients with lesions in this area of the dominant hemisphere will also be aphasic. A combination of verbal apraxia and Broca's aphasia is quite common [4]. Lesions of the right hemisphere rarely result in a significant apraxia; although some patients with right-hemisphere lesions have difficulty carrying out actions when asked to imitate the examiner [5].

Different types of apraxia have been categorized based on the complexity and nature of the task performed. The two major subgroups are *verbal* (apraxia of speech) and *nonverbal* apraxias. Verbal apraxia or apraxia of speech is an impairment in the ability to voluntarily produce speech. Nonverbal apraxia is an impairment in the ability to perform preplanned voluntary movements. Nonverbal apraxia can be further subdivided into *ideomotor* and *ideational* apraxia. In *ideomotor apraxia*, isolated gestures are impaired. This apraxia rarely affects spontaneous movements (such as waving good-bye) but is detectable in tasks in which the patient is asked to follow a verbal command or imitation. *Ideational apraxia* refers to a breakdown in performance of a task that involves a series of separate steps. It is usually seen in patients with bilateral brain disease. Ideational apraxia is generally associated with widespread intellectual deterioration, resulting in the patient's inability to effectively manipulate his or her environment (e.g., cooking a meal, lighting a cigarette, making a bed).

Constructional apraxia and dressing apraxia have also been described in the literature. *Constructional apraxia* is defined as an impaired ability to perform visuospatial tasks, such as drawing, assembling stick designs, and constructing three-dimensional block arrangements by verbal command or imitation. In dressing apraxia, the ability to dress oneself is lost. Both types of these apraxias are related to visuospatial difficulties in the dominant hemisphere.

Apraxia of Speech (Verbal Apraxia)

Apraxia of speech is commonly seen in combination with Broca's aphasia.

Lesion site: On or near the motor strip in the frontal lobe of the dominant hemisphere

Causes: Stroke, tumors, trauma

Characteristics

- Inconsistent errors
- Involuntary speech better than voluntary speech
- Struggles to untangle words

- Initial phonemes more in error than final phonemes
- Errors, including substitution, repetition, simplification, distortion, and addition
- Errors increase with word complexity
- Errors increase with word length
- Visual cues help patients
- More consonant than vowel errors
- Better accuracy with meaningful utterances than with nonmeaningful utterances

Ideational Apraxia

Ideational apraxia is usually seen in patients with bilateral brain disease or diffuse cortical disease. It is especially prominent in those diseases that affect the parietal lobes [1].

Lesion sites: Posterior parietal and temporoparietal lobes

Causes: Bilateral brain disease, diffuse cortical disease, stroke

Characteristics

- Inability to perform tasks that involve sequential steps (e.g., folding a piece of paper, putting it in an envelope, sealing it, addressing it, and placing a stamp on the letter) or everyday tasks such as making a bed
- Ability to perform the motor tasks in isolation
- Inability to recognize the use of objects (also called object agnosia)

Ideomotor Apraxia

Ideomotor apraxia is the most common type of apraxia.
Lesion sites: The premotor area, motor strip, or parietal or
temporal lobes in the dominant hemisphere [5, 6]
Causes: Stroke, trauma, tumor

Characteristics
- Inability to accurately perform previously learned
  motor acts

Types of Ideomotor Apraxia [5]
Buccofacial Apraxia (Oral Nonverbal Apraxia)
A test to determine oral apraxia is provided in Table 3.1.

Characteristics
- Disturbance of the volitional movements of the tongue,
  jaw, and lips during nonspeech tasks (e.g., whistling or
  drinking through a straw)
- May or may not occur with apraxia of speech
- Difficulty not due to muscle weakness or poor
  comprehension

Limb Apraxia
A test to determine limb apraxia is provided in Table 3.2.

Characteristics
- Inability to carry out acts on command, such as "Show
  me how you brush your hair" and "Show me how you
  hammer a nail."
- Ability to perform motor acts spontaneously

TABLE 3.1. Tests of isolated oral movement[a] and oral motor sequencing[b]

Isolated oral movement

Instructions: "I want you to make some movements with your lips, tongue, and jaw. Listen carefully and do just what I ask."

1. "Stick out your tongue."
2. "Try to touch your nose with your tongue."
3. "Try to touch your chin with your tongue."
4. "Bite your lower lip."
5. "Pucker your lips."
6. "Puff out your cheeks."
7. "Show me your teeth."
8. "Click your teeth together."
9. "Wag your tongue from side to side."
10. "Clear your throat."
11. "Cough."
12. "Whistle."
13. "Show that you are cold by making your teeth chatter."
14. "Smile."
15. "Show me how you would kiss a baby."
16. "Lick your lips."

Oral motor sequencing

Instructions: "Now, I want you to put some movements together. Watch me and do what I do."

1. Tongue (touch upper lip center)
   Jaw (lower and raise)
2. Teeth (click once)
   Lips (pucker)
3. Jaw (lower and raise)
   Teeth (bite lower lip)
   Lips (show teeth)
4. Tongue (touch lower lip center)
   Lips (pucker)
   Tongue (lick lips)
5. Lips (show teeth)
   Teeth (bite lower lip)
   Jaw (lower and raise)

TABLE 3.1. (continued)

> Tongue (lick lips)
> 6. Cheeks (puff out)
>   Lips (pucker)
>   Jaw (lower and raise)
>   Tongue (lick lips)
> 7. Teeth (click once)
>   Lips (pucker)
>   Jaw (lower and raise)
>   Tongue (lick lips)
>   Teeth (bite lower lip)
> 8. Lips (pucker)
>   Tongue (lick lips)
>   Teeth (click once)
>   Cheeks (puff out)
>   Tongue (touch upper lip center)

ᵃAdapted from WM Moore, JC Rosenbek, LL LaPointe. Assessment of Oral Apraxia in Brain-Injured Adults. In RH Brookshire (ed), Clinical Aphasiology: Conference Proceedings. Minneapolis: BRK Publishers, 1976;64.
ᵇAdapted from LL LaPointe, RT Wertz. Oral-movement and articulatory characteristics of brain-injured adults. Percep Mot Skills, 1974;39:39.
Source: RT Wertz, LL LaPointe, JC Rosenbek (eds). Apraxia of Speech in Adults: The Disorder and Its Management. San Diego: Singular, 1991;111.

- Difficulty not due to muscle weakness or poor comprehension

Apraxia of Whole Body Movements (Trunco-Pedal Apraxia)

Characteristics

- Difficulty with truncal commands, such as "Show me how you bow" and "Show me how you swing a baseball bat"

TABLE 3.2. Tests to determine the presence of limb apraxia

Instructions: "I want to see how you use your hands and arms to make some gestures. Listen carefully and do just what I ask."
  1. "Show how an accordion works."
  2. "Show me how you salute."
  3. "Wave good-bye."
  4. "Threaten someone with your hand."
  5. "Show that you are hungry."
  6. "Thumb your nose at someone."
  7. "Snap your fingers."
  8. "Show how you would play a piano."
  9. "Indicate that someone is crazy."
  10. "Make the letter 'O' with your fingers."

Source: RT Wertz, LL LaPointe, JC Rosenbek (eds). Apraxia of Speech in Adults: The Disorder and Its Management. San Diego: Singular, 1991;113.

MOTOR SPEECH EVALUATION

A motor speech evaluation is provided in Table 3.3 to help the examiner determine the presence of a motor speech disorder versus aphasic-type errors. This evaluation uses the multidimensional scoring system of the Porch Index of Communicative Ability provided in Table 3.4. Using this evaluation also helps the examiner distinguish an apraxia from a dysarthria. Once the presence of an apraxia has been established, its severity can be determined using Table 3.5. This table can also be used during the course of therapy to detect improvements in the patient's apraxia.

TABLE 3.3. Motor speech evaluation

Instructions: These test stimuli are to be recorded for patients suspected of demonstrating a motor speech disorder. Recording should be done at the standard loudness level using the standard microphone–patient distance. In each instance, elicit as adequate an attempt as the patient is capable of producing. Repeat and cue all ambiguous responses. For example, say to the patient, "Try it again. Say '_____,'" or "Watch me and do what I do." The cue for spontaneous speech is to continue asking questions. The cue for sentence imitation is to have the patient repeat one word at a time. The cue for the reading passage is to select one sentence, it does not matter which, and have the patient read each word as you point to it.

Scoring can be completed on the spot or from the tape and, depending on the purpose, can take a variety of forms:

1. A if apraxic, P if paraphasic, D if dysarthric, U if nondiagnostic error is observed, O if the error is other than above and specify what it seems to be (e.g., hearing), and N if normal.
2. Multidimensional: Use the Porch Index of Communicative Ability (PICA) multidimensional system (see Table 3.4), which is appropriate for all responses except for picture description and reading.
3. Transcription: Broad or narrow phonetic transcription at time of sample or after.

EVALUATION

1. Elicit five minutes of conversational speech according to the Boston Diagnostic Aphasia Examination method (see H Goodglass, E Kaplan. The Assessment of Aphasia and Related Disorders. Philadelphia: Lea & Febiger, 1984;4–5). Be sure to ask questions about illness, hospital stay, and speech and nonspeech symptoms.
2. "I want you to say '/a/' as long and evenly as you can. Like this '/a/'."
3. "Now, I want you to say some other sounds as long, as fast, and as evenly as you can."
   a. "Say '/p^-p^-p^/' as long, as fast, and as evenly as you can."
   b. "Say '/t^-t^-t^/' as long, as fast, and as evenly as you can."
   c. "Say '/k^-k^-k^/' as long, as fast, and as evenly as you can."
4. "Now, I want you to put three sounds '/p^/, /t^/, /k^/' together and say '/p^t^k^/' as long, as fast, and as evenly as you can. Like this, '/p^-t^-k^, p^-t^-k^, p^-t^-k^/'."

5. "Say these words for me as well as you can. You only have to say them once."
Gingerbread _____
Artillery _____
Snowman _____
Responsibility _____
Catastrophe _____
Television _____
Several _____
Tornado _____
Statistical analysis _____
Methodist Episcopal Church _____

6. "Now I want you to say these words after I say them. Repeat each word five times." (Score each production of each word.)
Artillery _____, _____, _____, _____, _____
Impossibility _____, _____, _____, _____, _____
Catastrophe _____, _____, _____, _____, _____

7. "Now, say these words after I say them."
Thick _____
Thicken _____
Thickening _____

Jab _____
Jabber _____
Jabbering _____

Zip _____
Zipper _____
Zippering _____

Please _____
Pleasing _____
Pleasingly _____

Flat _____
Flatter _____
Flattering _____

8. "Now, these."
Mom _____

TABLE 3.3. (continued)

Judge _____
Peep _____
Bib _____
Nine _____
Tote _____
Dad _____
Coke _____
Gag _____
Fife _____
Sis _____
Zoos _____
Church _____
Lull _____
Shush _____
Roar _____

9. "Say these sentences after me." (Cue is to give one word at a time with strong visual cue; record each production of each sentence.)
   The valuable watch is missing. _____
   In the summer they sell vegetables. _____
   The shipwreck washed up on the shore. _____
   Please put the groceries in the refrigerator. _____

10. "Count from one to twenty." (Score each production of each number.)

   1. _____
   2. _____
   3. _____
   4. _____
   5. _____
   6. _____
   7. _____
   8. _____
   9. _____
   10. _____
   11. _____
   12. _____
   13. _____
   14. _____

15. _____
16. _____
17. _____
18. _____
19. _____
20. _____

"Now, count backward from twenty to one." (Score each production of each number.)

20. _____
19. _____
18. _____
17. _____
16. _____
15. _____
14. _____
13. _____
12. _____
11. _____
10. _____
9. _____
8. _____
7. _____
6. _____
5. _____
4. _____
3. _____
2. _____
1. _____

11. "Tell me what is happening in this picture." (Elicit at least 1 minute of picture description from the patient based on the *Boston Diagnostic Aphasia Examination* "Cookie Thief" picture.)

12. "Repeat these sentences after me." (Use any four sentences the patient used spontaneously at any point in the evaluation. Write or transcribe the original [O] and the repetition [R]. Score each production of each sentence.)

    1.   O: _____
          R: _____
    2.   O: _____
          R: _____

TABLE 3.3. (continued)

3. O: _____
    R: _____
4. O: _____
    R: _____

13. "Now, read this passage out loud." (Have the patient read the "Grandfather Passage." Write or transcribe errors that may have diagnostic importance.) (See FL Darley, AE Aronson, JR Brown. Motor Speech Disorders. Philadelphia: Saunders, 1975;298 for the "Grandfather Passage.")

14. Summary

Diagnosis	Absent	Present	Suspected	Undetermined
Normal				
Aphasia				
Apraxia of speech				
Dysarthria (specify type)				
Language of confusion				
Language of generalized intellectual impairment				
Voice disorder (specify type)				
Other (specify)				

Source: Reprinted with permission from RT Wertz, LL LaPointe, JC Rosenbek (eds). Apraxia of Speech in Adults: The Disorder and Its Management. San Diego, CA: Singular, 1991;99.

DYSARTHRIA EXERCISES

Lip Exercises

1. Have the patient blot his or her lips firmly together and hold. Have the patient then relax. Have the patient repeat this process several times.

TABLE 3.4. Multidimensional scoring system of the Porch Index of Communicative Ability*

Score	Level	Description of response
16	Complex	Accurate, complex, and elaborate
15	Complex	Accurate and complete
14	Distorted	Accurate and complete but with reduced facility
13	Complete–delayed	Accurate and complete but slow or delayed
12	Incomplete	Accurate but incomplete
11	Incomplete–delayed	Accurate and incomplete but slow or delayed
10	Corrected	Accurate after self-correction of error
9	Repetition	Accurate after repetition of instruction
8	Cued	Accurate after cue or other information
7	Related	Inaccurate but related to correct response
6	Error	Inaccurate
5	Intelligible	Intelligible but not related to test item
4	Unintelligible	Unintelligible, differentiated
3	Minimal	Unintelligible, not differentiated
2	Attention	Attention to item but no response
1	No response	No awareness of test item

*The Porch Index of Communicative Ability multidimensional scoring system can be used to describe communicative responses in a therapeutic situation. This method of scoring is a way to reflect the subtle differences in a patient's language ability and can document subtle improvement throughout the course of recovery.
Source: Reprinted with permission from BE Porch. Porch Index of Communicative Ability: Theory and Development (Vol. 1). Austin, TX: PRO-ED, 1967.

2. Have the patient pucker his or her lips and hold. Have the patient relax. Have the patient repeat this process several times.

3. Have the patient say "oo-ee," exaggerating the movements with each production.

TABLE 3.5. Multidimensional scoring system to determine severity of apraxic patients

Score	Description
14	Normal
13	Normal, except slow because of changes in articulation and/or pause time
12	Normal, except for prosodic disturbance (pitch, loudness, stress, effort)
11	Distortion
10	Distortion and prosodic disturbance
9	Self-correction
8	Self-correction except for prosodic disturbance
7	Self-correction except for distortion
6	Groping that does not cross phoneme boundaries and is followed by the correct response
5	Sound substitution(s), omission(s), or addition(s), without sound distortion(s) or prosodic disturbances, but may have mild or moderate changes in articulation, pause time, or both Word remains recognizable
4	Sound substitution(s), omission(s), or addition(s) with distortion(s) or prosodic disturbances Word remains recognizable
3	Same as in 5 above except word is unrecognizable
2	Same as in 4 above except word is unrecognizable
1	No response, rejection, or unintelligible, undifferentiated response

Source: Adapted from M Collins, D Cariski, D Longstreth, et al. Patterns of Articulatory Behavior in Selected Motor Speech Programming Disorders. In RH Brookshire (ed), Clinical Aphasiology: Conference Proceedings. Minneapolis: BRK Publishers, 1980;196.

4. Have the patient say "oh" in an exaggerated motion with his or her mouth open.

5. Have the patient twist his or her mouth from left to right as if trying to stop his or her nose from itching.

6. Press the patient's bottom lip in a downward stroke with a tongue depressor. Have the patient try to resist having his or her lip pulled down. Repeat in an upward motion for the top lip.

7. Have the patient exaggerate a smile and hold it. Then have the patient relax. Have the patient repeat this process several times.

8. Have the patient repeat "may, me, my, mow, moo" several times.

9. Have the patient throw a kiss several times.

10. Have the patient puff his or her cheeks with air and hold the air for 5 seconds.

Tongue Exercises

General Tongue Exercises

1. Have the patient stick out his or her tongue and move it from corner to corner in the mouth.

2. Have the patient stick out his or her tongue as far as possible. Have the patient try to hold his or her tongue in the midline without any left or right deviation.

Tongue Tip Exercises

1. Have the patient stick out his or her tongue and try to touch his or her nose.

2. Have the patient say "la la la la."

3. Have the patient say "lay, lee, lie, low, lou." Have the patient repeat this sequence several times.

4. Have the patient press the tip of the tongue into his or her cheek, alternating from the left to the right side.
5. Ask the patient to stick out his or her tongue, and, using a tongue depressor, try to push his or her tongue back in his or her mouth. Have the patient try to resist.
6. Ask the patient to repeat "tic-tac-toe" slowly several times.

Posterior Tongue Exercises

1. Have the patient repeat "kitty cat" several times.
2. Have the patient repeat "cake, coke, kook" several times.
3. Have the patient press the back of his or her tongue to the roof of his or her mouth as if saying "/k/." Tell the patient not to let any air leak out his or her nose or mouth while holding this tongue position 1–2 seconds. Have the patient relax and then repeat this process five times.

Velar Exercises

1. Have the patient say "ah" sharply several times.
2. Have the patient directly stimulate his or her palate by touching it and coughing forcefully.

Exercises for Reduced Airway Closure

1. Have the patient hold his or her breath tightly while pushing or pulling on a chair. Have the patient repeat this process ten times.
2. Have the patient say "ah" while pushing against a chair. Have the patient repeat this process ten times.

3. Have the patient say "ah" with a hard glottal attack ten times.

4. Have the patient take a breath, hold it, then produce a strong cough. Repeat this process five times.

5. Have the patient practice coughing or clearing his or her throat. Have the patient repeat this process 10 times.

6. Beginning with the patient's head turned toward the stronger side, ask the patient to prolong an "ah" while slowly turning his or her head to the weaker side. At the point where production is interrupted, have the patient turn his or her head back to the stronger side and start again.

Exercises for Reduced Respiratory Support

1. Have the patient use a Voldyne/Triflo unit and gradually increase the target volume inspired.

2. Have the patient blow bubbles through a straw into a pitcher of water. Vary the depth of the straw to increase the difficulty.

3. Have the patient blow scraps of paper with a straw.

4. Have the patient sustain vowel and consonant sounds as long as he or she can and gradually try to increase the sustain.

5. Push against the patient's abdomen to assist weakened muscles as he or she sustains vowel sounds.

REFERENCES

1. Johns DF. Clinical Management of Neurogenic Communicative Disorders. Boston: Little, Brown, 1978;79, 251.
2. Aronson AE. Clinical Voice Disorders (3rd ed). New York: Thieme, 1990;77.
3. Prater RJ, Swift RW. Manual of Voice Therapy. Austin, TX: PRO-ED, 1984;125.
4. Marquardt T, Cannito M. Treatment of Verbal Apraxia in Broca's Aphasia. In G Wallace (ed), Adult Aphasia Rehabilitation. Boston: Butterworth-Heinemann, 1996;205.
5. Strub RL, Black FW. The Mental Status Examination in Neurology (3rd ed). Philadelphia: FA Davis, 1993;134.
6. Wertz RT, LaPointe LL, Rosenbek JC. Apraxia of Speech in Adults: The Disorder and its Management. San Diego: Singular, 1991;37.

SUGGESTED READING

Andrews ML. Manual of Voice Treatment: Pediatrics Through Geriatrics. San Diego: Singular, 1995.

Darley FL, Aronson AE, Brown JR. Motor Speech Disorders. Philadelphia: Saunders, 1975;298.

Goodglass H, Kaplan E. The Assessment of Aphasia and Related Disorders. Philadelphia: Lea & Febiger, 1984.

Love RJ, Webb WG. Neurology for the Speech–Language Pathologist (3rd ed). Boston: Butterworth-Heinemann, 1996.

Nicolosi L, Harryman E, Kresheck J. Terminology of Communication Disorders Speech-Language-Hearing (3rd ed). Baltimore: Williams & Wilkins, 1989.

Porch BE. Porch Index of Communicative Ability: Theory and Development. Auston, TX: PRO-ED, 1967.

4

Cranial Nerve Assessment

The 12 pairs of cranial nerves make up a part of the peripheral nervous system that transmits motor and sensory messages between the brain, head, and neck. Cranial nerve assessment can provide valuable information about the condition of the central nervous system, particularly the brain stem. The central nerves involved in speech and hearing are cranial nerves V (trigeminal), VII (facial), VIII (acoustic), IX (glossopharyngeal), X (vagus), and XII (hypoglossal) (Table 4.1).

TABLE 4.1. Cranial nerve assessment

Cranial nerve	Functions	Assessment	Disorders associated with cranial nerve lesions
I. Olfactory (sensory)	Smell	With the patient's eyes closed, occlude one nostril with your finger and ask the patient to identify smells (e.g., peppermint, gum, coffee, tea, cinnamon). Repeat the test on the other nostril.	Anosmia (loss of the sense of smell)
II. Optic (sensory)	Vision	Assess the patient's visual acuity with an eye chart. Ask the patient to count the number of fingers you hold up. To check visual fields, have the patient sit directly in front of you and stare at your nose. Slowly move your finger from the periphery toward the center until the patient says he or she can see it. Point at objects and ask the	Loss of vision

	Nerve	Function	Assessment	Abnormal findings
III.	Oculomotor (motor)	Innervation of muscles to move the eyeball Pupillary constriction Upper eyelid elevation	patient to tell you what color they are to check color vision. The motor functions of cranial nerves III, IV, and VI overlap; check them together by evaluating the patient's extraocular eye movement. Observe each eye for nystagmus, movement not in unison with that of the other eye, or the inability to move in certain directions. Note any complaint of double vision. To assess the oculomotor nerve, check pupil size, shape, and pupillary response to light.	Ptosis, diplopia, loss of accommodation, mydriasis
IV.	Trochlear (motor)	Innervation of superior oblique muscle of eye	See cranial nerve III (oculomotor)	Diplopia
V.	Trigeminal (sensory and motor)	Sensation to the face and head Corneal reflex Mastication Lateral jaw movements	To test motor function of the trigeminal nerve, have the patient clench his or her jaw, then try to separate the jaw.	Facial weakness and numbness

TABLE 4.1. (continued)

Cranial nerve	Functions	Assessment	Disorders associated with cranial nerve lesions
		To check for asymmetry, have the patient open and close his or her mouth.	
		To test sensory function, have the patient close his or her eyes, then lightly touch his or her forehead, cheeks, and jaw with a cotton ball. Have the patient indicate where he or she is being touched. Repeat this procedure using a sharp object, such as the cap of a ball-point pen.	
		Test the corneal reflex by lightly touching the patient's cornea with a cotton wisp.	
VI. Abducens (motor)	Abducts eye	See cranial nerve III (oculomotor)	Diplopia

VII. Facial (sensory and motor)	Movement of facial muscles Taste perception to anterior two-thirds of tongue Salivary glands	To test the motor portion, have the patient show his or her teeth, wrinkle his or her forehead, raise and lower his or her eyebrows, and puff out his or her cheeks. Have the patient close his or her eyes tightly while you gently attempt to open them with your hands. To test the sensory portion, have patient identify sugar, salt, lemon, and quinine swabbed on the anterior two-thirds of the tongue. Have patient identify flavors as sweet, salty, sour, or bitter. Alternate flavors and sides of the tongue. Have the patient rinse his or her mouth with water between flavors.	Upper and lower facial weakness, loss of taste for anterior two-thirds of the tongue, dry mouth, dysarthria
VIII. Acoustic (sensory)	Hearing Equilibrium	To test the acoustic portion of this nerve, test the patient's hearing acuity.	Vertigo, nystagmus, disequilibrium, deafness

TABLE 4.1. (continued)

Cranial nerve	Functions	Assessment	Disorders associated with cranial nerve lesions
		To test the vestibular portion, observe the patient's balance, and note complaints of dizziness. Observe for nystagmus.	
IX. Glossopharyngeal (motor and sensory)	Taste receptors to posterior one-third of tongue Sensations of throat Elevation of palate and larynx Salivary glands	Test the sensory portion at the same time as you assess CN VII, but apply the taste sensations to the posterior third of the tongue. CN IX and CN X have overlapping functions. Assess them together. Listen for hoarseness or nasality in the patient's voice. Observe soft palate elevation on "ah." Check gag reflex by touching the posterior pharyngeal wall with a cotton swab or tongue depressor.	Dysphagia, dysarthria, loss of taste for the posterior one-third of tongue, anesthesia of pharynx, dry mouth

X.	Vagus (sensory and motor)	Swallowing Gag reflex Phonation Taste Elevation of palate Activities of the thoracic and abdominal viscera Sensations of throat, larynx, thoracic, and abdominal viscera	See cranial nerve IX (glossopharyngeal)	Dysphagia, hoarseness, palatal weakness, cardiac dysfunction, dysfunctions of the viscera
XI.	Spinal accessory (motor)	Turning of head Shrugging of the shoulders	Palpate and inspect the sternocleidomastoid muscle as the patient attempts to turn his or her head to midline against resistance. Palpate and inspect the trapezius muscle as the patient shrugs his or her shoulders against your resistance.	Hoarseness, weakness of the head and shoulder muscles
XII.	Hypoglossal (motor)	Tongue movements	Observe the patient's tongue for asymmetry, atrophy, deviation to one side, and fasciculations.	Dysarthria, weakness or wasting of the tongue muscles

TABLE 4.1. (continued)

Cranial nerve	Functions	Assessment	Disorders associated with cranial nerve lesions
		Have the patient push the tip of his or her tongue against a tongue depressor and then ask the patient to try to push the depressor to one side and then the other. Have the patient first move his or her tongue rapidly from side to side with the mouth open, then curl the tongue up toward the nose, and finally curl his or her tongue down toward the chin. Listen for any distortion of the sounds /d/, /l/, /n/, and /t/.	

CN = cranial nerve.

Source: Adapted from IAC Golper. Sourcebook for Medical Speech Pathology. San Diego: Singular, 1992;132; S Loeb (ed). Illustrated Manual of Nursing Practice. Springhouse, PA: Springhouse, 1993;438; and RJ Love, WG Webb. Neurology for the Speech-Language Pathologist. Boston: Butterworth-Heinemann, 1992;112.

SUGGESTED READING

Golper LAC. Sourcebook for Medical Speech Pathology. San Diego: Singular, 1992.

Loeb S (ed). Nursing TimeSavers: Neurologic Disorders. Springhouse, PA: Springhouse, 1994.

Loeb S (ed). Illustrated Manual of Nursing Practice. Springhouse, PA: Springhouse, 1993.

Love RJ, Webb WG. Neurology for the Speech-Language Pathologist (3rd ed). Boston: Butterworth-Heinemann, 1996.

5

Cognitive Deficits

Cognition is a general term covering all the various modes of knowing: attending, perceiving, remembering, imagining, conceiving, judging, and reasoning [1]. Attention, language, and memory are the basic processes that allow for the development of higher intellectual abilities. When assessing a patient, his or her level of consciousness (LOC) should be established first. Next, the patient's ability to sustain attention over time should be determined before beginning to assess the more complex functions of memory, language, and abstract reasoning.

LEVELS OF CONSCIOUSNESS

A patient's LOC refers to the patient's ability to relate to himself or herself and his or her environment. Assessing a patient's arousal and awareness is necessary in determining the LOC. *Arousal* refers to the patient's ability to react to environmental stimuli, and *awareness* refers to his or her ability to correctly interpret the meaning of the stimuli. There are five levels (in order of most aroused to least aroused) clinicians use to distinguish LOC [2]:

Alertness   The patient is awake and fully aware of normal external and internal stimuli. The alert patient is able to interact with the clinician in a meaningful way.

Lethargy   The patient is not fully alert and tends to drift off to sleep when not actively stimulated. Spontaneous movements are decreased, and awareness is limited.

Obtundation   The patient is in a transitional state between lethargy and stupor. The patient is difficult to arouse and is confused when aroused. The patient usually requires constant stimulation.

Stupor and semicoma   The patient will respond only to persistent and vigorous stimulation. The patient cannot be roused spontaneously and is able only to groan or mumble and move restlessly when aroused.

Coma   The patient is completely unarousable. The patient does not respond to external or internal stimulation.

Neurologic disorders that may cause decreased levels of consciousness include brain tumor, cerebral aneurysm, cerebral contusion, cerebrovascular accidents, encephalitis, encephalomyelitis, encephalopathy, epidural hemorrhage, intracerebral hemorrhage, meningitis, pontine hemorrhage, seizure disorders, subdural hematoma, subdural hemorrhage, and transient ischemic attacks. Some nonneurologic causes for decreased levels of consciousness include: adrenal crisis, diabetic ketoacidosis, heatstroke, hyperglycemia, hypernatremia, hyperventilation syndrome, hypokalemia, hyponatremia, hypothermia, poisoning, shock, drug sedation, and alcohol use.

COMA SCALES AND THERAPY TECHNIQUES

The Glasgow Coma Scale (Table 5.1) provides an objective way to evaluate a patient's LOC and detect slight changes from the patient's baseline status. To determine the Glasgow Coma Scale score, add together the number of points from each section. A score of 3–4 indicates a deep coma with a poor prognosis and possible death. A score of 5–8 indicates that the patient has a severe brain injury. A score of 9–12 indicates that the patient has a moderate head injury. A score of 13–15 indicates that the patient has a mild head injury. Of the three components of the Glasgow Coma Scale, the motor response section yields the most useful prognostic information [3].

In comparison, the Rancho Levels of Cognitive Functioning Scale (Table 5.2) is very useful in helping therapists and families understand the behavior of each individual as he or she goes through rehabilitation. These levels apply specifically to patients suffering from head injuries during the first weeks or months after injury. These levels should not be used years later as a gauge of improvement [4].

It is important to note the differences between the Glasgow Coma Scale and the Rancho Levels of Cognitive Functioning Scale; the Glasgow Scale measures the levels of consciousness; the Rancho Scale measures postinjury behavioral responses (see Tables 5.1 and 5.2).

TABLE 5.1. Glasgow Coma Scale

Level of response	Appropriate stimulus	response	score
Eyes open	Approach to the bedside	Spontaneous	4
	Verbal command	Patient's eyes open to name.	3
	Pain	Patient does not open eyes in response to previous stimuli, but does to pain.	2
		None Patient does not open eyes in response to any stimulus.	1
Best motor response	Verbal command (e.g., "Raise your arm." "Hold up two fingers.")	Patient obeys commands.	6
	Painful stimulus	Patient pulls examiner's hand away when pinched. Patient finds offending stimulus and attempts to remove it.	5
		Patient pulls part of body away when it is pinched.	4
		Patient flexes body inappropriately to pain (decorticate posturing).	3

Level of response	Appropriate stimulus	Response	Score
		Patient's body becomes rigid in an extended position when pinched (decerebrate posturing).	2
		The patient has no motor response to pain.	1
Best verbal response	Score best verbal response when the patient is in his or her most alert stage.	The patient is oriented and converses. Patient knows who he or she is, where he or she is, and the year and month.	5
		The patient has confused conversation. Patient converses but is disoriented to either person, place, time, or date.	4
		Disorganized or inappropriate words without sustained conversation	3
		Incomprehensible Patient makes sounds but not recognizable words.	2
		None No sounds even with painful stimuli.	1

Source: Modified from B Jennett, G Teasdale. Assessment of Impaired Consciousness: Management of Head Injuries. Philadelphia: FA Davis, 1981.

TABLE 5.2. Rancho Levels of Cognitive Functioning Scale

Level I	No response stage
	No response to pain, touch, sound, or sight
Level II	Generalized response stage
	Limited, inconsistent, nonpurposeful responses, often to pain only
Level III	Localized response stage
	Blinks in response to bright light; turns toward or away from sound
	Responds to physical discomfort
	May focus on objects presented
	Responds inconsistently to commands
Level IV	Confused, agitated stage
	Confused, disoriented, agitated
	Alert, very active, with aggressive or bizarre behavior
	Unable to care for self
	Performs motor activities but behavior is nonpurposeful
	Unaware of present events
	Extremely short attention span
Level V	Confused, inappropriate, nonagitated stage
	Responds to commands
	Gross attention to environment, highly distractible, requires continual redirection
	Difficulty learning new tasks
	Agitated by too much stimulation
	May engage in social conversation but with inappropriate verbalizations
Level VI	Confused, appropriate stage
	Inconsistent orientation to time and place
	Retention span and recent memory impaired
	Begins to recall past
	Consistently follows simple directions
	Goal-directed behavior with assistance
Level VII	Automatic, appropriate stage
	Minimal confusion
	Performs daily routine in highly familiar environment in a non-confused, but automatic, manner
	Initiates tasks but needs structure

Skills noticeably deteriorate in unfamiliar environment

Poor judgment and problem-solving skills

Lacks realistic planning for own future, poor insight into condition

Level VIII   Purposeful, appropriate stage

Alert, oriented

Recalls past events

Learns new activities and can complete them without supervision

Independent in home and living skills

Persistent deficits in stress tolerance, judgment, and abstract reasoning

May function at a reduced level in society

Source: Reprinted with permission from C Hagen, D Malkmus, P Durham. Levels of Cognitive Functioning Scale. Downey, CA: Rancho Los Amigos Medical Center, Adult Brain Injury Service, 1980.

When working with a head-injured patient in the Rancho Levels of Cognitive Functioning, cognitive treatment techniques can be used to help plan treatment appropriate for the patient's level of functioning.*

The general goals of coma stimulation for a multidisciplinary team are the following:

To prevent sensory deprivation which can further depress impaired processing

To attempt to elicit responses that the patient may be capable of making

To increase cognition and motor responses

*The information is adapted from C Hagen. Language Disorders in Head Trauma. In A Holland (ed), Language Disorders in Adults. San Diego: College-Hill Press, 1984.

To attempt to heighten these responses and channel
them into meaningful activity
To normalize muscle tone
To maintain passive range of motion and prevent
contractures
To maintain skin integrity

The speech pathologist's role is to address the patient's cognitive deficits. Therapy sessions should begin with several 15-minute sessions and gradually increase to several 30-minute sessions. Basic skills should make up the primary goals initially to create a good foundation for higher cognitive skills. The hierarchy when selecting goals should progress from lower to higher skills as follows:

- Alertness
- Attention
- Selective attention
- Orientation
- Immediate memory
- Recent memory
- Organization
- Reasoning and problem solving
- Strategies to increase functional performance

The following levels correspond with the Rancho Cognitive Functioning Scale:

Level I   Unresponsive Stage

For a patient who is unresponsive, target all the sensory modalities.

Auditory Stimuli

- Play tape-recorded messages from friends and family members.
- Play favorite music or television show.
- Use bells and noise makers.

Visual Stimuli

- Show pictures of friends, family members, pets, or home.
- Show favorite items from home.
- Use clocks and calendars.
- Hang a mobile above the patient's bed with pictures of favorite items or foods.

Tactile Stimuli

- Brush different materials against the patient's skin (e.g., velvet, wool, cotton, satin).
- Brush or comb the patient's hair and talk about what you are doing.
- Wash the patient's face or hands.

Taste Stimuli

- Using cotton swabs, dab lemon, vinegar, and extracts on the patient's tongue.

Olfactory Stimuli

- Place containers of spices, soaps, and extracts beneath the patient's nose and talk about the smells. (Avoid the use of perfumes due to the possibility of allergic reactions.)

Level II   Generalized Responsiveness Stage

- Provide family education.
- Target arousal and attention.
- Continue environmental simulation as with Level I.
- Assess the patient's response to each stimulus one at a time. Try to elicit the same response with a different stimulus modality.
- Progress to getting the same response with a simple command, gesture, or tactile cue.
- When appropriate, assess the patient's swallowing and make recommendations.

Level III   Localized Response Stage

- Provide family education.
- Target reality orientation to self and the environment.
- Introduce yourself and explain what you are going to do, and then ask the patient to give the information back to you.
- Orient the patient to the environment.
- Continue environmental simulation as with Level I.
- Target the performance of simple commands.

Level IV   Confused-Agitated Stage

- Structure the environment to reduce stimuli and agitated behavior (e.g., decrease noise levels, decrease lighting, eliminate competing stimuli such as radios and televisions).
- Target increased attention to the environment.
- If it is indicated, train the patient with an augmentative communication system.
- Watch for impulsivity in the rate of eating and the amount of liquid or solids ingested per bite.
- Improve the length of attention by using simple cognitive tasks.
- Improve visual and auditory discrimination using simple language and cognitive tasks.
- Continue orientation therapy.
- Improve the patient's performance of simple verbal commands.
- When appropriate involve the patient's family in the therapy sessions.

Level V   Confused-Inappropriate Stage

- Work with the patient in a quiet environment; reduce the amount of visual and auditory stimuli.
- Avoid interruptions during the therapy session.
- Work on a basic set of orientation tasks daily (e.g., name, place, date, age, reason for hospitalization, etc.).
- Present tasks one at a time.
- Switch tasks if the patient becomes frustrated.

- Use concrete language.
- Encourage the patient to ask for clarification of instructions.
- Get eye contact before presentations and to monitor attention.
- Ask for feedback to check patient comprehension.
- Allow adequate response time.
- Do not argue with the patient or attempt to reason logically at this stage of recovery.
- Repeat correct responses without labeling the patient's response as wrong.

Level VI   Confused-Appropriate Stage

- Work on increasing the patient's responsiveness with minimal verbal cueing.
- Work on visual and auditory memory tasks and procedures (e.g., recall general idea of short paragraphs, word series, etc.).
- Begin to work on organizational skills (e.g., filling out shopping lists, listing the steps in a task, etc.).
- Begin to work on sequential tasks.
- Patient should begin to be able to carry over tasks learned from day to day.
- Patient should keep a daily log of events with assistance.

Level VII   Automatic-Appropriate Stage

- Work on developing higher cognitive skills (e.g., judgment, problem solving, insight, abstract reasoning, and detailed memory).

- Involve the patient in program planning, setting goals, and using leisure time.
- Involve the patient in simple activities of daily living (e.g., making his or her bed, light cleaning, light meal preparation).
- Work on complex activities that involve planning, memory for details, problem solving, and decision making.
- The patient should continue to keep a daily log of events.

Level VIII   Purposeful-Appropriate Stage

- The patient should be able to recall and integrate past and recent events.
- Continue work on abstract reasoning and judgment skills for emergencies or unusual situations.

MEMORY

Memory is a general term for the mental process that allows an individual to store information for recall at a later time. Memory loss may have an organic cause, such as Alzheimer's disease, acquired immunodeficiency syndrome (AIDS), herpes simplex encephalitis, head trauma, seizure disorders, frontal lobe tumors, and Korsakoff's syndrome. Not all memory disturbances are due to organic causes, however. Memory performance can also be impaired secondary to drug influences (see Appendix 5), anxiety, depression, alcoholic blackouts, electroconvulsive therapy, or hysteria [2, 5].

Memory can be divided into three basic types: *Immediate recall* (or *short-term memory*) refers to the recall of the past few seconds (such as the repetition of a series of numbers); *recent memory* refers to the patient's ability to learn and remember new material after a few minutes, hours, or days (such as recalling what was eaten for lunch); and *remote memory* refers to the ability to recall facts or events that occurred years before (such as historic facts or birth dates) [2].

Memory loss can be divided into two major types: *Retrograde memory loss* refers to amnesia for events that took place before the episode that caused the memory loss (e.g., head trauma), and *anterograde memory loss* refers to the inability to learn new material that occurs after the episode that caused the memory loss.

To quickly screen patients for disordered thought processes, you may ask the questions listed in Table 5.3. An incorrect answer to any question may indicate a need for a complete mental status evaluation. A good resource for a complete evaluation can be found in Strub and Black [1].

SIGNS AND SYMPTOMS FOR SENILE DEMENTIA OF THE ALZHEIMER'S TYPE

Millions of Americans suffer from some form of organic brain syndrome. Of those afflicted, approximately 50% have Alzheimer's disease, most of whom are older than age 65. (Nearly half of all North Americans older than age 85 have

TABLE 5.3. Mental status screening*

Question	Function screened
What is your name?	Orientation to person
How old are you?	Memory
When is your birthday? (month, day, year)	Remote memory
Where were you born?	Remote memory
Where are you right now?	Recent memory, location orientation
Why are you here?	Recent memory
What city are we in? (state, country)	Recent memory, location orientation
What is your address?	Recent memory, location orientation
What is today's date?	Recent memory, time orientation
What time is it right now?	Recent memory, time orientation
What season is it now?	Recent memory
What did you have for breakfast?	Recent memory
Who is the U.S. president?	Recent memory
Count backward from 20 to 1.	Attention and concentration

*Normal adults should have no difficulty answering these questions, although some normal adults will miss the exact date by 1 to 3 days, and the month. If a patient fails an item, tell the patient the correct answer, and have the patient repeat it. Retest the item several minutes later. If an incorrect response is again given, this indicates poor new learning abilities and will predict impairments on other memory tasks.
Source: Adapted from R Strub, FW Black. The Mental Status Examination in Neurology (3rd ed). Philadelphia: FA Davis, 1993;213.

Alzheimer's disease.) The remaining patients with organic brain syndrome have delirium and confusional states, amnesia syndromes, or non-Alzheimer's dementias [6].

Alzheimer's disease is the fourth leading cause of death in adults in the United States. Most patients die 2–15 years after the onset of symptoms. The average duration of the illness before death is 8 years.

Alzheimer's disease can be subdivided according to clinical stage, but there is great variability in the progression of the disease. It is not as orderly as the following descriptions imply, but these descriptions can be used as guidelines to help stage the disease [6, 7].

Early Stage of Senile Dementia of the Alzheimer's Type

Clinical Characteristics

- Recent memory loss
- Inability to learn and retain new information
- Word-retrieval problems
- Lability of mood
- Some change of personality possible
- Progressive difficulty performing activities of daily living (e.g., finding their way around, balancing a checkbook)
- Loss of ability to think abstractly
- Development of impaired judgment
- Irritability, hostility, or agitation
- Isolated aphasia or visuospatial difficulties

Intermediate Stage of Senile Dementia of the Alzheimer's Type

Clinical Characteristics

- Inability to learn or recall new information
- Becoming lost in familiar settings
- Significant risk for falls or accidents due to confusion

- Remote memory affected but not totally lost
- Assistance with activities of daily living required
- Uncooperativeness or physical aggressiveness
- Loss of sense of time and place

Severe or Terminal Stage of Senile Dementia of the Alzheimer's Type

<u>Clinical Characteristics</u>

- Inability to walk
- Total incontinence
- Complete dependency for all activities of daily living
- Possible inability to swallow
- Patient becomes mute
- Complete loss of recent and remote memory
- Eventual comatose state

TYPES OF DEMENTIAS

Some types of dementias are reversible. The potential for reversal exists when the cognitive deficits are related to drug toxicity, nutritional deficiencies, depression, normal pressure hydrocephalus, infection, cardiopulmonary disorders, or resectable brain lesions. Other types of dementias are irreversible. Irreversible types include Alzheimer's disease, Pick's disease, multi-infarct dementia, AIDS-related dementia, Creutzfeldt-Jakob disease, alcohol-related dementia, and cerebrocerebellar degenerations (such as Huntington's chorea) [2, 5].

Causes of Dementia

Irreversible dementia of an unspecified etiology
Alzheimer's disease
Vascular dementias
  Multi-infarct dementia
  Cortical microinfarcts
  Lacunar dementia
  Binswanger's disease
  Cerebral embolism
Degenerative diseases
  Pick's disease
  Parkinson's disease
  Huntington's disease
  Progressive supranuclear palsy
  Cerebellar degeneration
  Amyotrophic lateral sclerosis
  Multiple sclerosis
Specific infections
  Creutzfeldt-Jakob disease
  Progressive multifocal leukoencephalopathy
  Postencephalitic dementia
  Behçet's syndrome
  Acquired immunodeficiency syndrome
  Herpes encephalitis
  Neurosyphilis
  Fungal meningitis or encephalitis
  Bacterial meningitis or encephalitis
  Parasitic meningitis

Brain abscess
Trauma
    Dementia pugilistic
    Open or closed head injuries
Normal pressure hydrocephalus causing reversible and
    irreversible dementia
Autoimmune disorders
    Disseminated lupus erythematosus
    Vasculitis
Space-occupying lesions
    Primary brain tumor
    Chronic or acute subdural hematoma
    Metastatic tumors
Psychiatric disorders
    Depression
    Sensory deprivation
    Other psychoses
Drugs
    Sedatives
    Hypnotics
    Antianxiety agents
    Antidepressants
    Antiarrhythmics
    Anticonvulsants
    Digitalis
    Drugs with anticholinergic effects
Nutritional disorders
    Pellagra (vitamin B_{12} deficiency)
    Thiamine deficiency

Folate deficiency
Marchiafava-Bignami disease
Pernicious anemia
Metabolic disorders
Hyper- and hypothyroidism
Hypercalcemia
Hyper- and hyponatremia
Hypoglycemia
Hyperlipidemia
Hypercapnia
Cushing's syndrome
Addison's disease
Remote effect of carcinoma
Toxins
Alcoholic dementia
Metallic poisons (e.g., lead, mercury, arsenic, manganese)
Organic poisons (e.g., solvents, some insecticides)

REFERENCES

1. Nicolosi L, Harryman E, Kresheck J. Terminology of Communication Disorders: Speech, Language, Hearing (3rd ed). Baltimore: Williams & Wilkins, 1989;47.
2. Strub R, Black FW. The Mental Status Examination in Neurology (3rd ed). Philadelphia: FA Davis, 1993;30, 74, 213.
3. Jennett B, Teasdale G. Assessment of Impaired Consciousness. In B Jennett, G Teasdale (eds), Management of Head Injuries. Philadelphia: FA Davis, 1981;77.
4. Hagen C, Malkmus D, Durham P. Levels of Cognitive Functioning Scale. Downey, CA: Rancho Los Amigos Medical Center, Adult Brain Injury Service, 1980.

5. Golper LA. Sourcebook for Medical Speech Pathology. San Diego: Singular, 1992.

6. William B, Abrams MD, Berkow R (eds). The Merck Manual of Geriatrics. Rahway, NJ: Merck Sharp and Dohme Research Laboratories, Division of Merck and Co, 1990.

7. Reisberg B, Ferris SH, Leon MJ, Crook T. The global deterioration scale for assessment of primary degenerative dementia. Am J Psychiatry 1982;139:1136.

SUGGESTED READING

Hagen C. Language Disorders in Head Trauma. In A Holland (ed), Language Disorders in Adults. San Diego: College-Hill Press, 1984.

6

Dysphagia

Dysphagia refers to difficulty in swallowing. Swallowing difficulty can occur from a number of causes. Dysphagia is frequently associated with stroke, neurologic disease, and head and neck cancer surgery. In addition, swallowing problems sometimes occur with surgeries or disease processes that do not directly involve the oral, pharyngeal, or laryngeal structures. Aging can also cause dysphagia.

Table 6.1 lists of symptoms of dysphagia. Any of the symptoms, whether isolated or in combination, can be a sign of dysphagia. These behaviors do not necessarily indicate a swallowing disturbance, however. Objective studies are necessary to arrive at a definitive diagnosis. If your patient exhibits signs of a dysphagia, make a referral for a videofluoroscopic swallow study.

Patients who are experiencing dysphagia are at risk for malnutrition. Table 6.2 lists physical signs of malnutrition. These patients should be referred to a registered dietitian for a nutritional assessment. Table 6.3 lists other factors that can lead to malnutrition.

TABLE 6.1. Symptoms of dysphagia

Patient refuses food or avoids foods that require mastication.

Food spills from the patient's mouth during mastication.

Food remains in buccal pockets.

Patient eats slowly (more pronounced with solids).

Patient complains that "food won't go down" or that "food gets stuck."

Patient coughs, gags, or chokes before, during, or after a swallow.

Patient regurgitates food after meals.

Patient experiences nasal regurgitation.

Patient has a hoarse voice.

Patient experiences nasal or esophageal reflux.

Patient has a gurgly or wet vocal quality.

Patient complains of heartburn.

Patient has excessive secretions.

Patient drools.

Patient experiences excessive weight loss.

Patient's appetite is decreased.

X-ray reveals chronic lung changes.

Patient has frequent or recurrent pneumonia.

Patient has recurrent upper respiratory infections.

Infiltrates are noted on a chest x-ray, indicating some fluid density has built up in the lungs (usually located in the right middle lobe or right lower lobe of the lung).

Patient has frequent or recurrent low-grade fevers.

TABLE 6.2. Physical signs of malnutrition

- Dry, flaky skin
- Spoon-shaped nails
- Small yellowish lumps around the eyes
- Dull, dry hair
- Night blindness
- Gums that bleed easily
- Red, swollen lips
- Slow-healing wounds
- 5% weight loss in 1 month
- 10% weight loss of total body weight [4]
- Weight below 90% of the ideal [4]

TABLE 6.3. Factors that can lead to malnutrition

- Nothing by mouth or significantly reduced dietary intake for more than 3 days [4]
- Increased nutritional needs due to burns, trauma, infection, or surgery
- Increased nutritional needs due to disease processes (e.g., cancer, AIDS, coronary artery disease)
- Serum albumin <3.3 (see Appendix IV)
- Anorexia from illness or drug use
- Alcoholism or substance abuse
- Depression
- Dysphagia
- Chemotherapy and radiation therapy

ETIOLOGIES OF ASPIRATION

Aspiration occurs when any foreign substance penetrates the larynx and enters the airway below the true vocal folds. Aspiration pneumonia may result from infiltration of this foreign material into the lungs, particularly if the patient has an absent or weakened cough reflex. The main objectives of a swallowing evaluation are to determine if and why aspiration is occurring and to evaluate whether the aspiration can be cleared with a cough. Aspiration can occur at any of the swallowing stages. It can occur before the swallow due to reduced tongue control or a delayed or absent swallow reflex. Patients with neuromuscular weakness frequently have problems managing liquids and aspirate before the swallow. Aspiration can occur during the swallow due to reduced laryngeal closure or reduced laryngeal elevation. It can also occur after the swallow due to reduced tongue pressure on the bolus, reduced pharyngeal peristalsis, or cricopharyngeal dysfunction. Problems after the swallow usually involve semisolids or solids [1].

A patient who exhibits problems with any of the above but does not aspirate may still be at risk for aspiration when consuming large amounts of food or drink in an unsupervised eating situation. The patient may also be at risk if he or she has problems with lethargy or lack of alertness. In most patients with neurologic impairments, the sensitivity to aspiration is significantly reduced (Table

6.4). Many neurologically impaired patients are either unaware of their swallowing impairments or will deny any swallowing problem. Therefore, be aware of the potential for silent aspiration.

COMPENSATION AND TREATMENT FOR SWALLOWING PROBLEMS

When treating a dysphagic patient, the clinician must be sure exactly what he or she is treating. Swallowing therapy should not begin without an objective test and a definitive diagnosis. Although a bedside observation may give insight into a patient's disorder, it can lead to complications if the assessment is entirely subjective. Table 6.5 will assist the examiner in using the information gathered from a bedside evaluation and the radiologic findings to diagnose the patient experiencing dysphagia. Table 6.5 also provides compensatory strategies and treatment techniques appropriate for the different types of swallowing difficulties. Table 6.6 describes the various diet types available in a medical setting.

Specific compensatory strategies, such as the modified supraglottic swallow, and treatments, such as the modified Valsalva swallow, the Mendelsohn maneuver, and the Masako maneuver, may be required to ensure a patient can eat without aspirating. These techniques are described in detail in the next sections, as is the type of patient who can benefit from these techniques.

TABLE 6.4. Typical swallowing disorders in neurologic populations

I. Amyotrophic lateral sclerosis
Aspiration before the swallow due to reduced lingual control
Aspiration before the swallow due to a delayed swallowing reflex
Aspiration during the swallow due to reduced laryngeal closure
Aspiration after the swallow due to reduced pharyngeal peristalsis
Aspiration after the swallow due to cricopharyngeal dysfunction

II. Cerebellar degeneration
No consistent disorders

III. Cerebral palsy
Aspiration before the swallow due to reduced lingual control
Aspiration before the swallow due to a delayed swallowing reflex
Aspiration after the swallow due to poor pharyngeal peristalsis
Cricopharyngeal incoordination

IV. Head trauma
Aspiration before the swallow due to a delayed swallowing reflex
Aspiration after the swallow due to reduced pharyngeal peristalsis
Aspiration after the swallow due to cricopharyngeal dysfunction
Aspiration after the swallow due to a tracheoesophageal fistula
Reduced tongue control

V. Lateral medullary syndrome (Wallenberg's syndrome)
Cricopharyngeal dysfunction
Reduced pharyngeal peristalsis
Reduced laryngeal closure due to unilateral vocal cord paralysis

VI. Multiple sclerosis
Aspiration before the swallow due to reduced lingual control
Aspiration before the swallow due to a delayed swallowing reflex
Aspiration during the swallow due to reduced laryngeal closure
Aspiration after the swallow due to reduced pharyngeal peristalsis
Aspiration after the swallow due to cricopharyngeal dysfunction
Reduced pharyngeal peristalsis
Possible sensory changes

VII. Myasthenia gravis
Involvement of any cranial nerve musculature
Fatigue

VIII. Myotonic dystrophy
Aspiration after the swallow due to cricopharyngeal dysfunction

IX. Oculopharyngeal dystrophy
    Reduced pharyngeal peristalsis
 X. Parkinson's disease
    Abnormal lingual peristalsis
    Reduced pharyngeal peristalsis
    Delayed reflex
    Reduced laryngeal closure
    Cricopharyngeal dysfunction
XI. Stroke (cortical and brain stem)
    Aspiration before the swallow due to a delayed swallowing reflex
    Aspiration during the swallow due to reduced laryngeal closure (usu-
        ally in brain stem strokes)
    Aspiration after the swallow due to reduced pharyngeal peristalsis
    Aspiration after the swallow due to cricopharyngeal dysfunction
    Disrupted lingual peristalsis

Source: Modified from J Logemann. Evaluation and Treatment of Swallowing Disorders. San Diego: College-Hill, 1983.

The Modified Supraglottic Swallow

The modified supraglottic swallowing technique is used in cases of inadequate airway protection mechanisms when aspiration is documented or a high risk. It is particularly indicated when a patient is known to be a silent aspirator. Have the patient follow these steps:

1. Use a cut-out cup or remove one-third of a side of a Styrofoam cup to prevent the patient's nose from hitting the rim of the cup during the swallow. This also helps to prevent neck extension, thus opening the airway.

TABLE 6.5. Bedside and radiographic symptoms of dysphagia and their causes and treatments

Bedside symptom	Radiographic finding	Possible cause	Compensation and treatment
Holding food in mouth Inability to initiate a swallow Delayed elevation of the hyoid bone and thyroid cartilage	Hesitation of material in the vallecular sinus before initiating the swallowing reflex	Delayed swallowing reflex	Diet change to thickened liquids and pureed foods Use of cold or stimulating pureed foods (e.g., sour or spicy) Thermal stimulation Tilting the head down Applying quick, downward pressure to the tongue 3-sec preparation (the patient consciously pauses to organize the bolus transfer and elicit a swallow) "Slurp and swallow" (patient places bolus centrally in his or her oral cavity, then slurps or sucks the bolus into the phar-

Bedside symptom	Instrumental examination	Possible cause	Management
			ynx, followed promptly by elicitation of a swallow)
Food falls out of the mouth	Same as bedside symptom	Poor lip closure	Lip exercises
Drooling, lower lip retraction, and facial asymmetry	Same as bedside symptom	Damage to cranial nerve VII; Decreased labial strength; Accumulation of oral residue	Applying short, rapid, downward strokes to the edge of the bottom lip, emphasizing the affected side, using a cool washcloth just before each meal and again at the end of the meal; Oral-facial exercises; Tilting head to unaffected side; Oral hygiene
Food remaining in mouth or spilling from mouth; Buccal pocketing of food	Material spreads throughout the oral cavity; Material falls into the sulci	Loss of oral sensation	Ingesting only cool or warm foods; Verbal cues to swallow; Oral hygiene; Lingual sweep; Use of a mirror to cue the patient when food is spilling and during oral hygiene; Consecutive swallows

TABLE 6.5. (continued)

Bedside symptom	Radiographic finding	Possible cause	Compensation and treatment
Absent or prolonged oral preparation	Same as bedside symptom	Cognitive impairment Sensory or motor impairment Salivary gland hypofunction Reduced oral awareness	Verbal cues to chew and swallow
Material spreads throughout the mouth	Loss of bolus control, material spreads throughout the oral cavity Material falls over the base of tongue into the valleculae or the airway and is aspirated before the swallow		Diet change to thickened liquid Use of cold or stimulating foods Alternating bites of cold foods with those of other temperatures Lingual sweep
Coughing or choking before the swallow	Aspiration before the swallow Material spills over from the sinuses into the airway prior to the swallow	Reduced tongue coordination Delayed swallow reflex (bolus enters pharynx before a swallow is initiated)	Diet change to thickened liquids Neck flexion Tongue exercises 3-sec preparation (conscious pause to allow patient to organize bolus transfer and elicit a swallow) Supraglottic swallow

Slow oral transit time Food catches in mouth Food residue on hard palate	Slow oral transit time Reduced tongue elevation Collection of material on hard palate	Reduced tongue elevation	Tongue exercises
Slow oral transit time Eating is more difficult with solids	Slow oral transit time Repeated pumping motion of the tongue	Reduced or disorganized anterior to posterior tongue movement	Tongue exercises Neck extension posture (if the risk of aspiration is not present)
Slow oral transit time	Slow oral transit time Collection of material in tongue depression from scarring, worsening with tongue movement	Scarred tongue contour	Effortful swallow Supraglottic swallow Positioning of food
Cannot chew or avoids foods requiring mastication; material remains midline on tongue or falls into sulcus	Material remains midline on tongue or falls into sulcus	Reduced lateral tongue movement	Soft diet Tongue exercises Oral hygiene
Pocketing of food in cheeks	Material falls into sulcus	Reduced buccal tension Poor tongue control Impaired oral sensation	Tilting of head to the stronger side Lingual sweep Cheek exercises Placing food on the stronger side Applying pressure on outside of cheek

TABLE 6.5. (continued)

Bedside symptom	Radiographic finding	Possible cause	Compensation and treatment
Food residue in mouth after swallow	Loss of bolus control Material spreads throughout oral cavity Material falls over base of tongue into the vallecular sinus or airway before the swallow	Reduced tongue control	Diet change to chopped, ground, or pureed foods and thickened liquids Placing food on posterior of tongue Tongue exercises Tilting the head back
Coughing after food or fluids	Aspiration after the swallow Pharyngeal pooling	Delayed or absent swallow reflex	Diet change to thickened liquids and pureed foods Placing food on the strongest side of the mouth Neck flexion or chin tuck posturing Avoiding straws Modified supraglottic swallow "Dry" swallows Use of a cut-out cup
Nasal voice quality Inability to suck	Poor velar elevation	Poor velar elevation	Velar strengthening exercises

Symptom	Site of residue	Cause	Intervention
Wet, gurgly vocal quality	Pyriform sinus residue Spillover of material to level of vocal cords		Palatal lift Alternating solids and liquids Neck flexion or chin tuck posturing Double swallows after each bite Volitional cough or throat clearing after every 2 or 3 bites
Nasal burning or dripping	Reflux into nasal cavity	Reflux of food into the nasal cavity due to poor elevation of the velum Often related to injury of cranial nerves IX, X, and XII	Avoiding acidic and carbonated foods and liquids Exercises that enhance velum elevation
Burning or tickling at the back of the throat	Residue in vallecular sinus	Usually related to food or medication pocketing in the vallecular sinus	Sitting the patient at at least a 60-degree angle before administering anything orally Placing crushed pills in applesauce or ice cream Double swallows after each bite to clear

TABLE 6.5. (continued)

Bedside symptom	Radiographic finding	Possible cause	Compensation and treatment
			pharynx and assist peristaltic action
			Turning head to the weaker side
Coughing, choking, or observable decreased laryngeal elevation	Aspiration after the swallow Reduced thyroid elevation	Reduced laryngeal elevation	Supraglottic swallow Modified Valsalva swallow Pitch exercises and use of falsetto "Dry" swallows Neck flexion or chin tuck posturing Mendelsohn maneuver
Coughing or choking during the swallow Hoarseness	Aspiration during the swallow Reduced vocal cord adduction	Reduced laryngeal closure	Adduction exercises, forceful phonation, coughing, clearing the throat Supraglottic swallow Tilting head forward Pitch exercises and use of falsetto Effortful swallows Mendelsohn maneuver
Food sticks high in the	Residue of material on	Unilateral pharyngeal	Turning head to the

throat	one side of valleculae or one pyriform sinus	dysfunction	weaker side Tilting head to the stronger side
Food expectorated after the swallow	Residue of material in the vallecular or the pyriform sinuses after the swallow	Reduced pharyngeal peristalsis	Alternating liquids and solids Limiting size of bites "Dry" swallows Falsetto modified Valsalva maneuver
Coughing or choking after the swallow Gargling vocal quality Excessive secretions	Aspiration after the swallow due to spillover from pyriform sinus Collection of material in pyriform sinus	Cricopharyngeal dysfunction	Liquid or semisolid diet Mendelsohn maneuver
Bad taste in mouth upon waking or excessive burping	Esophageal reflux	Esophageal reflux	Sitting upright during meals Sitting up for 1 hr after each meal Drinking a carbonated beverage before bedtime Elevating head of bed at night
Patient complains of food sticking in the lower throat	Collection of material in the cervical esophagus after the swallow	Reduced esophageal peristalsis	Alternating liquids and solids

TABLE 6.5. (continued)

Bedside symptom	Radiographic finding	Possible cause	Compensation and treatment
Leaving half of the food on a tray untouched	N/A	Visual field deficit	Verbal and tactile cueing to remind the patient to scan the tray
Long eating sessions	Poor bolus control and mastication	Fatigue Poor bolus control, mastication, or swallowing skills High distractibility	Frequent meals with less food Verbal cueing Exercises to improve mastication
Short eating sessions	N/A	Motor ataxia Impulsivity usually associated with right brain damage	Spacing of food presentation Pacing techniques Verbal cueing Medical intervention
Regurgitation of food Coughing or choking after the swallow	Collection of material in a side pocket in the pharynx or esophagus Failure of food to pass through the esophagus	Esophageal diverticulum	Medical intervention
Regurgitation of food Coughing or choking after the swallow	Aspiration after the swallow from esophageal overflow	Partial or total obstruction in pharynx or esophagus	Medical intervention

| Coughing or choking after the swallow | Material passes from esophagus into trachea | Tracheoesophageal fistula | Medical intervention |
| Material leaks out hole onto skin | Material leaks through skin | Pharyngocutaneous fistula | Medical intervention |

Source: Modified from J Logemann. Evaluation and Treatment of Swallowing Disorders. San Diego: College-Hill, 1983; and B Emick-Herring, P Wood. A Team Approach to Neurologically Based Swallowing Problems in Rehabilitation Nursing (Vol. 15, No. 3). Skokie: IL, Association of Rehabilitation Nurses, 1990;126.

TABLE 6.6. Diet types

Diet type	Description
Clear liquid diet	Water, clear fruit juices, clear broth, gelatin, tea, and coffee
Full liquid diet	Liquid and strained fruit juices, milk, ice cream, gelatin, tea, and coffee
Pureed diet	Foods that require no chewing and are easy to swallow (similar to full liquid diet, but includes pureed fruits, vegetables, and meats)
Mechanical soft diet	Foods that require little or no mastication (ground meats, well-cooked, easy-to-chew fruits and vegetables)
Dysphagia diet	Pureed fruits, vegetables, and meats, and thickened liquids
Regular diet	Standard diet for patients without special dietary needs
Prescribed therapeutic diets	Special needs diets (e.g., low-sodium, diabetic diet)
Bland diet	Eliminates foods that have been shown to cause gastrointestinal irritation, flatus, or bloating; foods are mildly spiced and low in acidity; indicated for patients who are immobilized
Soft diet	Similar to a regular diet; the foods are tender but not ground or pureed; high-fiber foods are omitted

2. Have the patient hold his or her breath before and during the swallow. While the patient holds his or her breath, have the patient take a bolus in the mouth, flex the neck, and tuck the chin against his or her chest.

3. Have the patient continue holding his or her breath with the neck flexed and the chin tucked. Have the patient swallow the bolus. (Repeated swallows may be necessary to clear the oral cavity and pharynx.)

4. After the swallow and before inhaling, the patient coughs to clear any residue from the top of the airway [1, 2].

Mendelsohn Maneuver

The Mendelsohn maneuver is used with patients who have reduced laryngeal elevation and pharyngeal contraction, or with those who have hypertonicity of the cricopharyngeal sphincter.

1. Have the patient swallow, and feel the rise of his or her larynx.

2. Have the patient swallow again and prolong the tongue contraction. This will prolong the elevation of the larynx.

Masako Maneuver

The Masako maneuver is used with patients who have weakened posterior pharyngeal wall contraction or with patients who have poor base-of-tongue-to-pharyngeal-wall approximation [3].

1. Anchor the patient's tongue anteriorly. This may be done by holding the tongue tip with gauze.

2. Have the patient "dry" swallow with the tongue in this forward position. The posterior pharyngeal wall should begin to come forward to compensate. (This maneuver should not be done using a food or liquid.)

Modified Valsalva Swallow

This treatment is used with patients who have decreased laryngeal elevation and pharyngeal contraction. Patients with cardiac conditions should have medical clearance before using this technique.

1. The patient should sit with both feet firmly on the floor.

2. Have the patient swallow "hard" (as if swallowing a large piece of food).

REFERENCES

1. Logemann J. Evaluation and Treatment of Swallowing Disorders. San Diego: College-Hill, 1983;37, 127, 211.
2. Emick-Herring B, Wood P. A Team Approach to Neurologically Based Swallowing Problems in Rehabilitation Nursing (Vol. 15, No. 3). Skokie, IL: Association of Rehabilitation Nurses 1990;126.
3. Fujiu M, Logemann JA. Effects of a tongue-holding maneuver on posterior pharyngeal wall movement during deglutition. Am J Speech-Lang Pathol 1996;5:22.
4. Groher ME. Dysphagia: Diagnosis and Management (2nd ed). Boston: Butterworth-Heinemann, 1992;255.

SUGGESTED READING

Golper LC. Sourcebook for Medical Speech Pathology. San Diego: Singular, 1992.

O'Gara JA. Dietary adjustments and nutritional therapy during treatment for oral-pharyngeal dysphagia. Dysphagia 1990;4:209.

7

Diagnostic Tests
of the Nervous System

The tests discussed in this chapter assist in the diagnosis of
the major disorders of the brain and its cavities, vasculature, and coverings; the brain stem and cranial nerves; the
spinal cord and spinal roots; and the peripheral nerves and
the major skeletal muscle groups they innervate.

When treating patients with stroke, neuromuscular
disease, brain tumors, or other neurologic disorders, the
clinician can obtain information from these tests. Such
information can help the clinician to confirm a speech
diagnosis and to make treatment decisions, as well as
provide prognostic information.

CEREBRAL ANGIOGRAPHY

Cerebral angiography provides radiographic examination
of the cerebral vasculature after injection of a contrast
medium [1, 2].

Purpose

- To detect disruption or displacement of the cerebral circulation by aneurysm, arteriovenous malformation, hemorrhage, thrombosis, narrowing, or occlusion
- To study vascular displacement caused by tumor, hematoma, edema, herniation, vasospasm, increased intracranial pressure, or hydrocephalus
- To locate clips applied to blood vessels during surgery and to evaluate the postoperative status of such vessels

CEREBROSPINAL FLUID ANALYSIS

Cerebrospinal fluid (CSF) for analysis is most often obtained by lumbar puncture. In rare cases, it is obtained by cisternal or ventricular puncture [1, 2].

Purpose

- To measure CSF pressure to detect an obstruction of CSF circulation
- To aid diagnosis of viral or bacterial meningitis, subarachnoid or intracranial hemorrhage, tumors, and brain abscesses
- To aid diagnosis of neurosyphilis and chronic central nervous system (CNS) infections

DIGITAL SUBTRACTION ANGIOGRAPHY

Digital subtraction angiography is a sophisticated radiographic technique that uses video equipment and computer-assisted image enhancement to examine the vascular systems. X-ray images are obtained after injection of a contrast medium [2, 3].

Purpose

- To detect and evaluate cerebrovascular abnormalities (e.g., carotid stenosis and occlusion, arteriovenous malformations, aneurysms, and vascular tumors)
- To visualize extracranial and intracranial cerebral blood flow in order to view displacement of vasculature by other intracranial pathology or trauma
- To detect lesions often missed by computed tomography (CT) scans
- To aid postoperative evaluation of cerebrovascular surgery such as arterial grafts and endarterectomies

ELECTROENCEPHALOGRAPHY

Electroencephalography (EEG) produces a record of the brain's electrical activity through the placement of electrodes on standard areas of the patient's scalp [2, 3].

Purpose

- To detect reduced electrical activity in an area of cortical infarction
- To differentiate seizure activity from cerebrovascular accident (CVA)
- To determine the presence and type of epilepsy
- To aid diagnosis of intracranial lesions (e.g., abscesses and tumors)
- To evaluate the brain's electrical activity in metabolic disease, head injury, meningitis, encephalitis, mental retardation, and psychological disorders
- To confirm brain death

ELECTROMYOGRAPHY

Electromyography (EMG) is the recording of the electrical activity of selected skeletal muscle groups at rest and during voluntary contraction. It is a diagnostic technique for evaluating muscle disorders [2, 3].

Purpose

- To aid in differentiating between primary muscle disorders (e.g., the muscular dystrophies) and secondary muscle disorders
- To assist in the diagnosis of diseases characterized by central neuronal degeneration (e.g., amyotrophic lateral sclerosis)

- To aid in the diagnosis of neuromuscular disorders (e.g., myasthenia gravis)

EVOKED POTENTIAL STUDIES

Evoked potential studies evaluate the integrity of visual, somatosensory, and auditory nerve pathways by measuring the brain's electrical response to stimulation of the sense organs or peripheral nerves [2, 3].

Purpose
- To diagnose nervous system lesions and abnormalities
- To assess neurologic function
- To monitor comatose patients and patients under anesthesia
- To evaluate the neurologic function in infants whose sensory systems cannot be adequately assessed
- To monitor spinal cord function during spinal cord surgery

Visual Evoked Potentials

Visual evoked potential studies are used to evaluate the integrity of the visual nerve pathways by exposing the eye to a rapidly reversing checkerboard pattern.

Purpose
- To evaluate demyelinating disease
- To evaluate traumatic injury
- To evaluate visual complaints

Somatosensory Evoked Potentials

To measure somatosensory evoked potentials, electrodes are attached to the patient's skin over somatosensory pathways to stimulate peripheral nerves.

Purpose

- To diagnose peripheral nerve disease (e.g., Guillain-Barré syndrome, multiple sclerosis)
- To locate brain and spinal cord lesions

Auditory Evoked Potentials

Auditory evoked potentials are produced by delivering clicks to the ear and measuring the brain's response to the stimulation.

Purpose

- To locate auditory lesions
- To evaluate brain stem integrity

INTRACRANIAL COMPUTED TOMOGRAPHY

Intracranial CT provides a series of tomograms, translated by a computer and displayed on a monitor, that represent cross-sectional images of various layers of the brain. This technique can reconstruct cross-sectional, horizontal, sagittal, and coronal plane images. Intracranial tumors and other brain lesions may be identified as areas of altered density.

Tissue densities appear as white, black, or shades of gray, with the densest tissue appearing white and the least dense tissue appearing black. Bone appears white. Ventricular and subarachnoid CSF appear black. Brain matter appears in shades of gray. Structures are evaluated according to their density, size, shape, and position. Intracranial CT scanning may eliminate the need for painful and hazardous invasive procedures, such as pneumoencephalography and cerebral angiography [2, 3].

Purpose

- To diagnose intracranial lesions and structural abnormalities (e.g., tumors, hematomas, cerebral atrophy, nonhemorrhagic infarction, aneurysms, edema, or congenital anomalies such as hydro-cephalus)
- To monitor the effects of surgery, radiotherapy, or chemotherapy on intracranial tumors
- To assess focal neurologic abnormalities and other clinical features that suggest an intracranial mass
- To provide early diagnosis of subdural hematoma in a patient with suspected head injury before it causes characteristic symptoms

MAGNETIC RESONANCE IMAGING

Magnetic resonance imaging (MRI) produces highly detailed cross-sectional images of the brain and spine in multiple planes. It can scan through bone and delineate fluid-filled soft tissue. MRI is useful in the diagnosis of cerebral infarction, tumors, abscesses, edema, hemorrhage, nerve fiber demyelination, and other disorders that increase the fluid content of affected tissues. MRI can show irregularities of the spinal cord and produce images of organs and vessels in motion. No harmful side effects have been documented [2, 3].

Purpose
- To aid in the diagnosis of intracranial and spinal lesions and soft-tissue abnormalities
- To evaluate the location and size of lesions

MYELOGRAPHY

Myelography combines fluoroscopy and radiography to evaluate the spinal subarachnoid space after injecting a contrast medium. It can help locate a spinal lesion, a ruptured disk, spinal stenosis, or an abscess [2, 3].

Purpose
- To reveal lesions, such as tumors and herniated intervertebral disks, that partially or totally block the flow of CSF in the subarachnoid space
- To aid in the detection of arachnoiditis, spinal nerve root injury, or tumors in the posterior fossa of the skull

OCULOPLETHYSMOGRAPHY

Oculoplethysmography is a noninvasive procedure that indirectly measures blood flow in the ophthalmic artery. Since the ophthalmic artery is the first major branch of the internal carotid artery, its blood flow accurately reflects carotid blood flow and that of cerebral circulation [3].

Purpose

- To aid in the detection and evaluation of carotid occlusive disease

POSITRON EMISSION TOMOGRAPHY

Positron emission tomography (PET) provides images of detailed brain function and brain structure through sophisticated computer reconstruction algorithms. PET measures the emission of injected radioisotopes and coverts these to a tomographic image of the brain.

Purpose

- To evaluate cerebral blood flow changes
- To pinpoint sites of glucose metabolism

SKULL RADIOGRAPHY

Skull radiography is a noninvasive neurologic test that involves taking x-ray films of the skull.

Purpose

- To detect fractures in head trauma patients
- To aid in the diagnosis of pituitary tumors
- To detect congenital and perinatal anomalies

- To aid in the diagnosis of systemic diseases that produce bone defects of the skull

TENSILON TESTS

Tensilon tests involve careful observation of the patient after intravenous administration of edrophonium chloride (Tensilon). Tensilon is a rapid, short-acting anticholinesterase that improves muscle strength by increasing muscular response to nerve impulses. It is especially useful in diagnosing myasthenia gravis [2, 3].

Purpose
- To aid in the diagnosis of myasthenia gravis
- To aid in differentiation between myasthenic and cholinergic crises
- To monitor oral anticholinesterase therapy

TRANSCRANIAL DOPPLER STUDIES

Transcranial Doppler studies measure the velocity of blood flow through cerebral arteries. These studies provide information about the presence, quality, and changing nature of circulation to an area of the brain [2, 3].

Purpose
- To measure the velocity of blood flow through certain cerebral vessels
- To help detect arteriovenous malformations

- To detect and monitor the progression of cerebral vasospasm
- To determine whether collateral blood flow exists before surgical ligation or radiologic occlusion of diseased vessels
- To help determine brain death

OTHER TESTS TO DIAGNOSE CEREBROVASCULAR ACCIDENTS

The following tests help identify causes of CVAs.

Doppler Ultrasonography

Doppler ultrasonography evaluates blood flow in the major veins and arteries of the arms and legs and in the extracranial cerebrovascular system [1–3].

Purpose

- To examine the size of the intracranial vessels and the direction and velocity of cerebral blood flow
- To aid in the diagnosis of chronic venous insufficiency and superficial and deep vein thromboses
- To aid in the diagnosis of peripheral artery disease and arterial occlusion
- To monitor patients who have had arterial reconstruction and bypass grafts
- To detect abnormalities of carotid artery blood flow associated with such conditions as aortic stenosis
- To evaluate possible arterial trauma

Electrocardiography

Electrocardiography reveals abnormalities caused by a cardiac-induced CVA.

Purpose

- To help identify primary conduction abnormalities, cardiac arrhythmias, cardiac hypertrophy, pericarditis, electrolyte imbalances, myocardial ischemia, and the site and extent of myocardial infarction (MI)
- To monitor recovery from MI
- To evaluate the effectiveness of cardiac medication
- To assess pacemaker performance

Magnetic Resonance Angiography

Magnetic resonance angiography (MRA) is a recent development in the field of magnetic field technology. MRA is more expensive than conventional angiography and does not represent a replacement technology. It is a noninvasive technique that helps determine the need for conventional angiography [2].

Purpose

- To provide images of cerebral blood vessels
- To help determine whether conventional angiography is needed

Ophthalmoscopic Examination

Ophthalmoscopic examination allows magnified examination of the vascular and nerve tissue of the fundus, including the optic disk, retinal vessels, macula, and retina [1].

Purpose

- To detect hypertension and atherosclerotic changes in retinal arteries
- To detect and evaluate eye disorders as well as ocular manifestations of systemic disease

Single-Photon Emission Computed Tomography

Single-photon emission computed tomography (SPECT) tracks radioisotopes, allowing detection of perfusion defects in patients with CVA before there is CT evidence of infarction and during transient ischemic attacks.

Purpose

- To identify cerebral blood flow
- To diagnose cerebral infarction

REFERENCES

1. Loeb S (ed). Nursing TimeSavers: Neurologic Disorders. Springhouse, PA: Springhouse, 1994;185.
2. Shaw M (ed). Professional Handbook of Diagnostic Tests. Springhouse, PA: Springhouse, 1995;495, 567, 619.
3. Loeb S (ed). Illustrated Guide to Diagnostic Tests. Springhouse, PA: Springhouse, 1994;759

8

Laryngeal Cancer

Laryngeal cancer is a malignant growth on the vocal cords or other parts of the larynx. Squamous cell carcinoma accounts for approximately 95% of all cases of laryngeal cancer. The other 5% is made up of rare forms of cancer such as adenocarcinoma and sarcoma [1].

The exact cause of laryngeal cancer is not known. Major risk factors include cigarette smoking and alcoholism. Minor risk factors include chronic inhalation of noxious fumes, genetic predisposition, and a history of laryngitis and vocal straining [1].

Accurate identification of the site of the tumor is important, since the spread of malignancy is directly related to tumor location. Tumors on the true vocal cords do not spread because the underlying connective tissue lacks lymph nodes. Tumors of this type have a very good prognosis for complete removal. Tumors on the other parts of the larynx, however, tend to spread rapidly.

The tumor, node, metastasis system was developed by the American Joint Committee on Cancer for the purpose of staging laryngeal cancer (Table 8.1). The system divides the larynx into three regions—supraglottis, glottis, and sub-glottis. The supraglottis is composed of the epiglottis (suprahyoid epiglottis and infrahyoid epiglottis), aryte-noepiglottic folds, arytenoids, and false vocal cords. The glottis is composed of the true vocal cords, including the anterior and posterior commissures. The subglottis is the region extending from the lower boundary of the glottis to the lower margin of the cricoid cartilage [2].

Malignant tumors of the larynx are usually character-ized by the following:

- Average age of occurrence is between 50 and 70 years
- Usually associated with cigarette smoking, alcohol use, or both
- Vocal hoarseness (usually the first sign)
- Possible inhalatory stridor
- Possible lump in the neck or throat
- Throat pain
- Shortness of breath
- Possible difficulty swallowing
- Weight loss
- Possible ear pain
- Cough

TABLE 8.1. Staging of laryngeal cancer

Primary tumor (T)

TX	Primary tumor cannot be assessed
T0	No evidence of primary tumor
Tis	Carcinoma in situ

Supraglottis

T1	Tumor limited to one subsite of supraglottis, with normal vocal cord mobility
T2	Tumor invades more than one subsite of supraglottis or glottis, with normal vocal cord mobility
T3	Tumor limited to larynx with vocal cord fixation and/or invades postcricoid area, medial wall of pyriform sinus, or pre-epiglottic tissues
T4	Tumor invades through the thyroid cartilage and/or extends to other tissues beyond the larynx (e.g., to the oropharynx or soft tissues of neck)

Glottis

T1	Tumor limited to vocal cord(s) (may involve anterior or posterior commissures), with normal mobility
T1a	Tumor limited to one vocal cord
T1b	Tumor involves both vocal cords
T2	Tumor extends to supraglottis, and/or subglottis, and/or with impaired vocal cord mobility
T3	Tumor limited to the larynx, with vocal cord fixation
T4	Tumor invades through thyroid cartilage and/or extends to other tissues beyond the larynx (e.g., oropharynx or soft tissues of neck)

Subglottis

T1	Tumor limited to the subglottis
T2	Tumor extends to vocal cord(s), with normal or impaired mobility
T3	Tumor limited to larynx, with vocal cord fixation
T4	Tumor invades through cricoid or thyroid cartilage and/or extends to other tissues beyond the larynx (e.g., oropharynx or soft tissues of neck)

TABLE 8.1. (continued)

Regional lymph nodes (N)

NX	Regional lymph nodes cannot be assessed
N0	No regional lymph node metastasis
N1	Metastasis in a single ipsilateral lymph node, ≤3 cm in greatest dimension
N2	Metastasis in a single ipsilateral lymph node, >3 cm but not >6 cm in greatest dimension; or metastasis in multiple ipsilateral lymph nodes, none >6 cm in greatest dimension; or metastasis in bilateral or contralateral lymph nodes, none >6 cm in greatest dimension
N2a	Metastasis in a single ipsilateral lymph node >3 cm but not >6 cm in greatest dimension
N2b	Metastasis in multiple ipsilateral lymph nodes, none >6 cm in greatest dimension
N2c	Metastasis in bilateral or contralateral lymph nodes, none >6 cm in greatest dimension
N3	Metastasis in a lymph node >6 cm in greatest dimension

Distant metastasis (M)

MX	Presence of distant metastasis cannot be assessed
M0	No distant metastasis
M1	Distant metastasis

Staging grouping

Stage 0	Tis	N0	M0
Stage I	T1	N0	M0
Stage II	T2	N0	M0
Stage III	T3	N0	M0
	T1	N1	M0
	T2	N1	M0
	T3	N1	M0
Stage IV	T4	N0	M0
	T4	N1	M0
	Any T	N2	M0
	Any T	N3	M0

	Any T	Any N	M1

Histopathologic grade (G)

GX	Grade cannot be assessed
G1	Well differentiated
G2	Moderately differentiated
G3	Poorly differentiated
G4	Undifferentiated

Source: Reprinted with permission from the American Joint Committee on Cancer, AJCC Manual for Staging of Cancer (4th ed). Philadelphia: Lippincott-Raven, 1992;39.

SURGICAL OPTIONS FOR LARYNGEAL CANCER

Endoscopy with Laser Surgery

- Endoscopy with laser surgery is an option if tumor is confined to a small area, usually to one true vocal cord.
- This procedure is performed during laryngoscopy.
- A laser beam is used to remove or reduce the size of the glottic tumor.
- The voice is preserved after surgery.

Transoral Cordectomy [1]

- Transoral cordectomy is performed during laryngoscopy.
- This procedure is used to resect an early, small tumor limited to the true vocal cords.
- The voice is preserved after surgery.
- Prognosis for complete removal of the cancer is good.

Laryngofissure [1]

- Laryngofissure is used to remove larger glottic tumors confined to a singe vocal cord.
- Prognosis for complete removal of the cancer is good.
- The patient will have a temporary tracheostomy after surgery.
- The patient's voice may be hoarse initially after surgery.

Vertical Hemilaryngectomy [1, 3]

- Vertical hemilaryngectomy is used to remove widespread laryngeal cancer.
- The surgeon removes about one-half of the thyroid cartilage and the subglottic cartilage, one false vocal cord, and one true vocal cord and then rebuilds the area with the strap muscles.
- The patient will have a temporary tracheostomy after surgery.
- The patient will be hoarse initially after surgery.
- The patient will have continued vocal roughness, breathiness, and decreased volume after surgery.
- The patient may experience some temporary difficulty with aspiration during the swallow after surgery.
- The patient should not receive thin liquids initially after surgery.
- Have the patient flex the neck forward and tuck the chin to reduce the risk of aspiration.

- Postsurgical concerns include teaching the patient swallowing compensation techniques, and control of voice quality, reducing vocal hyperfunction and phrase length, and increasing the patient's vocal fold closure.

Horizontal Supraglottic Laryngectomy [1, 3]

- Horizontal supraglottic laryngectomy is used to remove a large supraglottic tumor.
- The surgeon removes the epiglottis, aryepiglottic folds, hyoid bone, part of the thyroid cartilage, and false vocal cords.
- The true vocal cords are not removed.
- A cricopharyngeal myotomy is usually performed to facilitate swallowing.
- The patient will have a temporary tracheostomy after surgery.
- The patient retains his or her voice after surgery.
- The patient will have vocal roughness, reduced vocal range, and reduced volume after surgery.
- The patient may have dysphagia after surgery, with aspiration during the swallow.
- Teach the patient a supraglottic swallow or voluntary airway protection technique to help prevent the possibility of aspiration that occurs after the surgery is performed.
- Postsurgical concerns include dysphagia management, vocal cord abuse reduction, increasing intelligibility, and minimizing vocal roughness.

Near Total Laryngectomy [4]

- Near total laryngectomy preserves the voice in selected patients with advanced laryngeal lesions.
- Resection includes the entire larynx except for a narrow strip connecting the trachea and the pharynx over an uninvolved arytenoid cartilage.
- Posterior true and false vocal cords and the hemisubglottis on the uninvolved side are preserved.
- A tracheoesophageal shunt is formed over the remaining tissue, and the remainder of the pharyngeal wall is closed primarily.
- The patient is able to vocalize through the shunt after surgery.
- The patient is permanently tracheotomy-dependent after surgery.
- The patient will have temporary dysphagia after surgery.
- Postsurgical concerns include dysphagia management and training the patient to coordinate breathing and voicing.

Total Laryngectomy [1]

- Total laryngectomy is used to remove a large glottic or supraglottic tumor attached to the vocal cord.
- The surgeon removes the true vocal cords, false vocal cords, epiglottis, hyoid bone, cricoid cartilage, and two or three tracheal rings.
- The surrounding tissue may also need to be removed.
- The patient will have a permanent tracheostomy and a laryngeal stoma after surgery.

- The patient's natural voice is lost after surgery.
- See the section on postoperative consultation for laryngectomy for postsurgical concerns.

Radical Neck Dissection or Selective Neck Dissection [1]

- Radical neck dissection or selective neck dissection is used when cancer has spread to surrounding tissues and glands.
- The surgeon extends the supraglottic or total laryngectomy to remove the cervical chain of lymph nodes, the sternocleidomastoid muscle, the fascia, and the internal jugular vein on the side of the tumor.
- The patient will temporarily lose range of motion in one shoulder after surgery.
- This surgery disfigures the patient.
- See the section on postoperative consultation for laryngectomy for postsurgical concerns (Figures 8.1 and 8.2).

PRE- AND POSTOPERATIVE CONSULTATION FOR LARYNGECTOMEES

Preoperative Consultation for Laryngectomy

Before making a preoperative visit with a patient, consult with the physician about what information he or she would like you to address. Many physicians believe that the patient should be informed, but not burdened with so much information that it causes increased anxiety. Many

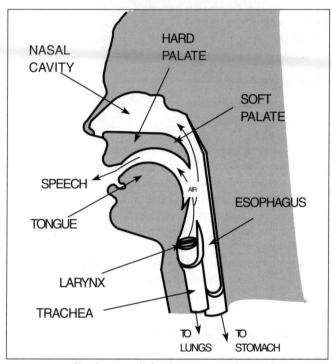

Figure 8.1. Profile of a person before laryngectomy, showing basic anatomy of the neck and airways.

times, the stress of impending surgery interferes with a patient's ability to absorb the information discussed in the preoperative meeting. With this in mind, it may be a good

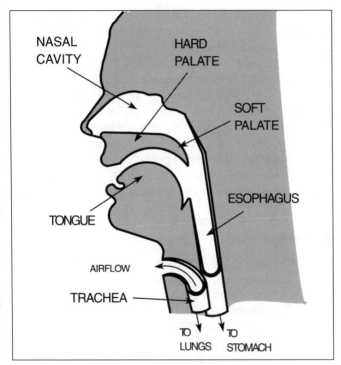

Figure 8.2. Profile of a person after laryngectomy, showing the basic anatomic and physiologic changes that occur as a result of this procedure.

idea to limit the initial preoperative visit to introducing yourself and defining your role as the clinician that will assist the patient in restoring his or her communication after surgery. Obtain medical, occupational, educational, and social history. During your conversation, make an informal observation as to the patient's dialect, articulation patterns, and overall intelligibility. Have literature from the American Cancer Society or the International Association of Laryngectomees to leave for the patient and family members to read. Explain that you will be happy to answer any questions they may have at a later date. Be optimistic and reassuring to your patient. The information that follows may be more beneficial if discussed postoperatively. Once again, deciding what issues to address is a decision to make with the attending physician.

Postoperative Consultation for Laryngectomy

I. Review: Be prepared to review any or all of the preoperative consultation information discussed with the patient.
II. Communication options after surgery
    A. Types of artificial larynx devices
        1. Neck model
        2. Tube-in-the mouth model
        3. Pneumatic artificial larynx devices
        4. Dental-appliance model
    B. Esophageal speech concerns
        1. Patient will need an initial insufflation test.
        2. To become proficient requires several months of speech therapy.

C. Tracheoesophageal voice prosthesis
1. Primary puncture (If the patient is punctured during surgery, full voice should not be used for about 12–14 days.)
   a. No additional surgery is required.
   b. Patient avoids the nasogastric tube after surgery and is fed directly into the red rubber catheter.
   c. There is no risk. If the patient is unable to produce voicing the doctor will remove the catheter, and the puncture will heal in a few hours.
2. Secondary puncture
   a. The procedure can be done months or years after the laryngectomy surgery.
   b. The patient must wait 3–6 months after the total laryngectomy before he or she can have surgery again.
   c. Insufflation testing should be done prior to surgery to determine if tracheoesophageal (TE) speech is possible.
   d. Patient must wait at least 6 weeks from the time of the puncture to the time of the fitting.
III. Support organizations
A. Local chapters of the Lost Chord Club
B. Local chapters of the American Cancer Society
C. Hospital family support groups

       D. International Association of Laryngectomees (see Appendix I: National Support Groups and Informational Organizations)

IV. Physical changes the patient can expect (Be prepared to show the patient pictures that illustrate the anticipated changes.):

    A. Stoma used for breathing and coughing

    B. No longer will breathe through mouth or nose

    C. Decreased sense of smell

    D. Decreased sense of taste

    E. Decreased ability to lift due to inability to perform Valsalva maneuver

    F. Increased difficulty in having a bowel movement due to inability to perform Valsalva maneuver

V. What the patient can expect immediately after surgery (A patient may be experiencing anxiety about the hospital equipment or his or her physical status after surgery.):

    A. Placement of an intravenous tube

    B. Use of a suction tube

    C. Placement of a Hemovac to drain excess blood and other fluids

    D. Placement of laryngectomy tube to keep the stoma open initially

    E. Use of oxygen equipment

    F. Excessive secretions from stoma

    G. Feeding tube for several days

    H. Pain

    I. Initial difficulty swallowing after a diet is begun

    J. Liquid diet

    K. Depression

    L. Communication through writing or gestures

    M. Physical therapy if a radical neck dissection is performed

    N. Speech therapy follow-up to begin electrolarynx training if indicated

VI. Safety issues

    A. The patient will need a smoke detector in his or her home.

    B. The patient will need to purchase an emergency medical identification bracelet, which identifies the patient as a neck breather in case of the need for emergency cardiopulmonary resuscitation.

    C. The patient should not go swimming.

    D. The patient should keep the stoma covered at all times.

    E. The patient should avoid smoke, paint fumes, powders, sprays, and other irritants.

    F. The patient should use a rubber shower shield to prevent water from entering the stoma while bathing.

VII. Stoma care

    A. The speech pathologist or nurse should instruct the patient on the use of saline to thin stoma secretions.

    B. The patient should wash his or her hands before handling the stoma.

C. The patient should clear the airway by coughing before going to bed and after waking up.

D. The patient should clean the area around the stoma with warm water.

E. The patient should not use paper tissue or cotton balls to clean the stoma because they can be aspirated.

F. If crusting occurs around the stoma, the patient should moisten with water, wait, and then wipe away crust or use tweezers to remove it.

G. The patient should not use oils or lotions as lubricants. The patient should use K-Y Jelly or some other water-soluble lubricant to lubricate the edges of the stoma.

H. The patient should use a humidifier in the home.

VIII. Helpful aids and devices

A. Humidifilters

B. Voice amplifiers

C. Emergency medical identification bracelets

D. Emergency identification

E. Plastic stoma buttons

F. Stoma covers

G. Shower collars

IX. Possible postoperative complications (**Discuss these only as the problems arise.** There is no reason to increase the patient's anxiety if these problems never occur.)

A. Follow-up radiation therapy can create any of the following problems:
   1. Cause skin breakdowns
   2. Make learning esophageal speech more difficult
   3. Make the healing process take longer
   4. Make swallowing more difficult
B. Swallowing difficulties
   1. Tracheoesophageal fistula—breakdown of tissue between the trachea and the esophagus allowing food to enter the trachea (Coughing or choking should not occur when the patient eats or drinks after surgery. If this happens the patient should notify the physician at once.)
   2. Pharyngoesophageal stricture—scar tissue that narrows the esophagus and prevents a large bolus or a bolus of thick consistency from passing through the esophagus
   3. Pseudoepiglottis—scar tissue band at the base of the tongue that forms a pocket where food and liquid collect during the swallow
C. Stenosis of the stoma
   1. Stoma ideally should be the size of a quarter or nickel.
   2. If stenosis occurs
      a. Patient should notify the physician

     b. Modification of the stoma site may be
       required
     c. Patient may need to wear a stoma button

DYSPHAGIA IN ORAL AND LARYNGEAL CANCER PATIENTS

Patients with resected oral structures typically have difficulty with mastication, forming and controlling the bolus, and moving the bolus to the back of the mouth for swallowing. Patients who lose up to a third of their tongue have transitory swallowing disorders. Patients who undergo a glossectomy that includes the base of the tongue are more likely to have persistent dysphagia, but the majority can successfully learn to eat orally.

Partial Tongue Resection [3]

Problems That Can Occur When Less Than 50% of the Tongue Is Removed

- Temporary dysphagia
- Difficulty triggering the swallowing reflex

Problems That Can Occur When More Than 50% of the Tongue Is Removed

- Decreased lingual peristalsis
- Decreased control of the bolus

Therapeutic Interventions

- Thermal stimulation

- Tongue exercises (see the section on dysphagia exercises after surgery or radiation treatment for oral cancer)
- Head tilted back for swallowing
- Voluntary airway protection (supraglottic swallow technique)

Anterior Floor of Mouth Composite Resection [3]

Problems

- Reduced labial closure
- Aspiration before the swallow due to reduced lingual control
- Temporary delayed swallowing reflex
- Difficulties with lingual control of the bolus, lingual peristalsis, and mastication

Therapeutic Interventions

- Food positioned more posteriorly on the tongue
- Head tilted back for swallowing
- Pureed diet
- Voluntary airway protection (supraglottic swallow technique)
- Tongue exercises (see the section on dysphagia exercises after surgery or radiation treatment for oral cancer)

Tonsil or Base of Tongue Composite Resection [3]

Problems

- Reduced tongue range of motion
- Aspiration before the swallow due to reduced lingual control
- Aspiration before the swallow due to a delayed swallow reflex
- Aspiration after the swallow due to reduced pharyngeal peristalsis
- Nasal regurgitation if extended to the soft palate

Therapeutic Interventions

- Tongue exercises to increase range of motion (see the section on dysphagia exercises after surgery or radiation treatment for oral cancer)
- Therapy to improve the triggering of the swallow reflex (see Chapter 6, Table 6.5)
- Voluntary airway protection (supraglottic swallow technique; see Chapter 6)

Hemilaryngectomy [3]

Problems

- Temporary difficulty with aspiration
- Aspiration during the swallow due to reduced airway closure if extended

Therapeutic Interventions

- Flex head forward for swallowing
- Vocal fold adduction exercises (see the section on dysarthria exercises in Chapter 3)

Supraglottic Laryngectomy (Subtotal Horizontal Laryngectomy) [3, 5]

Problems

- Aspiration during the swallow due to reduced laryngeal closure
- Aspiration after the swallow due to reduced pharyngeal peristalsis

Therapeutic Interventions

- Use of supraglottic swallow technique (see Chapter 6)
- Vocal fold adduction exercises (see Chapter 3)

Total Laryngectomy [3]

Problems

- Pseudoepiglottis
- Pharyngoesophageal stricture
- Tracheoesophageal fistula

Therapeutic Interventions

- Medical intervention required

• Prior to dilation of the pharyngoesophageal stricture, change of diet to liquid or pureed foods

Pharyngeal Resection

Problems

• Aspiration after the swallow due to reduced peristalsis

Therapeutic Interventions

• Double swallows per bolus (see Chapter 6, Table 6.5)
• Alternating liquids and solids

Radiation Therapy to the Oral Cavity and Neck [3]

Problems

• Reduced saliva production (xerostomia)
• Edema
• Mouth sores
• Aspiration before the swallow due to a delayed swallowing reflex
• Aspiration after the swallow due to reduced peristalsis

Therapeutic Interventions

• Double swallows per bolus (see Chapter 6, Table 6.5)
• Alternating liquids and solids
• Thermal stimulation

- Provide patient with information about saliva substitution products on the market

Mandibulectomy

Problems

- Interference with mastication
- Lengthened oral phase of the swallow
- Poorly timed bolus propulsion, delayed propulsion, or both

Therapeutic Interventions

- Range of motion exercises to improve jaw movement (see the section on dysphagia exercises after surgery or radiation treatment for oral cancer)
- Soft diet
- Three-second preparation swallow (see Chapter 6, Table 6.5)

Total Glossectomy with Tracheostomy

Problems

- No bolus manipulation
- Poor bolus propulsion

Therapeutic Interventions

- "Dump" swallow technique (Pureed food is placed in a large gauged syringe. While the patient's head

is tilted back with his or her mouth open, the syringe is placed in the posterior oral cavity and emptied.)
• Selection of alternative communication device

Glossectomy and Submental Resections [3]

Problems

• Decreased tongue propulsion
• Decreased lip sensation
• Decreased protective tilting action of the larynx
• Significant aspiration

Therapeutic Interventions

• Clinician-controlled tongue manipulation of a large object such as a large button tied to a string
• Range of motion exercises for the tongue (see the section on dysphagia exercises after surgery or radiation treatment for oral cancer)

DYSPHAGIA EXERCISES AFTER SURGERY OR RADIATION TREATMENT FOR ORAL CANCER

Oral Sensory Stimulation of the External (Facial) Area

1. Using a cotton swab, lightly tap from midline laterally, inferiorly, and superiorly over impaired facial regions, including lips, cheeks, chin, and nares.

2. Using your fingertips, apply a light, rapid, circular motion with gentle stretch, and massage the patient's impaired facial areas.

3. Alternate light and firm touches to the patient's lips, cheeks, and chin using fingers, a cotton swab, or a small spoon.

4. Stimulate the patient's facial region, alternating cold (ice chips in a plastic bag) and warm (wash cloth).

Oral Sensory Stimulation of the Internal (Oral) Area

1. Clean the patient's oral cavity. Gently apply circular motion to all oral areas using a cotton swab dipped in lemon juice. Repeat until the patient elicits some perception of touch.

2. Touch a spot in the patient's mouth with a cotton swab, and have the patient move his or her tongue to the same spot. Apply light pressure as the tongue touches the target spot with the swab.

3. Touch the patient's cheek with your finger and have the patient touch the corresponding spot inside his or her cheek with his or her tongue. Apply pressure from the outside as the tongue touches the spot inside the mouth.

4. Using a swab, touch the oral structures and verbally describe the location as you proceed from front to back and side to side. Repeat until the patient has an image of the internal borders of his or her reconstructed oral cavity.

5. Identify an internal oral location to the patient, and have the patient move his or her tongue to that point without tactile or visual cues.

Lip Motion, Strength, and Contact

1. Have the patient use his or her fingers to tap and massage around the mouth.

2. Have the patient use his or her fingers to round and retract his or her lips.

3. Have the patient attempt voluntary unaided rounding and retracting of the lips using a mirror to monitor motions.

4. Place three to five tongue depressors between the patient's lips. Exert upward and downward pressure gently and encourage any active motion or resistance. Remove one tongue depressor at a time and repeat to increase strength.

5. Have the patient use wide-rimmed cups to encourage lip contact. Have the patient move these in and out of the mouth rapidly and then slowly to stimulate lip motion and to achieve closure. Use a spoon in a similar manner when the patient is able.

6. Actively or passively have the patient maintain lip closure. Have the patient pucker his or her lips forcefully and attempt to suck in. (The patient may need to inhale.) Stroking the patient's chin or neck may aid sucking response.

7. Have the patient hold a piece of thick plastic tubing between his or her lips. Have the patient suck air through the tube. Hold the tube in place as needed. Reduce the size and length of tubing to create a better seal, and have the patient try to suck.

8. Use a straw in the same fashion as the tube, occluding the open end as the patient sucks in.

Tongue Strength and Motion

See Chapter 3 for tongue strength and motion exercises.

Velar Exercises

See Chapter 3 for velar exercises.

Chewing and Jaw Exercises

1. Place wet gauze squares between the patient's molars. Have the patient bite down and use his or her tongue to move the gauze squares between the molars on the right side and chew.

2. Place gauze on the patient's lips, and have the patient practice forming a bolus and moving it into position to chew.

3. Use manual manipulation to help patient make mandibular and maxillary molar contact on intact side of mouth. Place your hand on the patient's jaw while he or she chews the gauze on the opposite side. When the patient is successful with the gauze, use a piece of gum.

4. Have the patient move his or her jaw from side to side with the mouth closed.

5. Have the patient close his or her mouth. Apply downward pressure on the patient's chin while the patient resists opening his or her mouth.

6. Have the patient open his or her mouth. Push up on the patient's jaw as the patient resists closing his or her mouth.

SELECTING THE BEST ALARYNGEAL SPEAKING METHOD FOR A PATIENT

Esophageal speech is generally considered the most desirable alaryngeal communication option. Although it requires training, after it is mastered, there are no further expenses involved, no parts to maintain, and no hassles with additional surgery or closing of puncture sites. Unfortunately, not every laryngectomy patient is capable of achieving esophageal speech. Successful air intake for esophageal speech is dependent on appropriate tension of the upper esophageal sphincter. This can be determined with a simple insufflation test before beginning any esophageal training (see the section on insufflation testing). If the patient fails the insufflation testing and still desires this communication option, a pharyngeal constrictor myotomy or a pharyngeal plexus neurectomy will be required (see the section on myotomies and neurectomies).

Patients who desire or require a proficient method of immediate communication after total laryngectomy (e.g., a patient who must return quickly to work) should consider a tracheoesophageal puncture (TEP). A TEP does not prevent using regular esophageal speech or an artificial larynx. Once again, not every patient is a candidate for this procedure (see the section on TEP for the established guidelines for determining TEP candidates). The TEP works well for many, but some patients do not have the necessary strength or tissue structure. Some patients have continual problems with infection, respiratory diseases, candidiasis, tissue tearing, or coughing the device out of place. Maintenance of a TEP requires good eyesight, hand coordination, and the mental ability to properly care for it. The development of prostheses that may be worn for several months at a time is making these points less of an issue, however.

Most laryngectomy patients will probably need either temporary or permanent access to an artificial larynx. Esophageal speech takes time to develop, and candidates for a secondary puncture will have to wait several months for the follow-up surgery. An artificial larynx is also useful for proficient esophageal speakers in times of illness or for TEP patients suffering from a respiratory illness or an infection of the puncture. It is also useful if there is a need for repuncture or stoma revision. Many doctors and speech-language pathologists recommend that an artificial larynx be kept on hand to use at night, during illness, or in an emergency.

Patients who require an immediate method of communication but do not meet the requirements for TEP or esophageal speech training will need to consider purchasing an artificial larynx. See the section on selecting an artificial larynx to determine the best model for the patient.

Laryngectomy patients who have multiple problems (e.g., very radical neck surgery, total glossectomy, or both in combination with the total laryngectomy, loss of tongue control, or stroke or head injury resulting in aphasia, dysarthria, or apraxia) may have to rely on a communication board or computer adaptation. These devices range from simple picture cards to sophisticated computers with choices of voice, print, or liquid crystal display. QWERTY, alphabet, symbol, or picture orientation systems are available. Systems may be operated by keyboards, touch pads, single switch input, or eyegaze. For communication options contact the Augmentative and Alternative Communication Journal. (See Appendix I, National Support Groups, for the phone number and address.)

Selecting an Artificial Larynx

When deciding on which artificial larynx is best suited for the patient, take into consideration the patient's physical coordination, intelligence and cognitive ability, ability to follow directions, eyesight, health and cleanliness habits, and any substance addictions. People who are alcoholic or have excessive secretions may have difficulty keeping food, beverages, and medications from getting down the tube of an intraoral device, causing corrosion. Patients who have difficulty keeping their hands clean or dry will need to choose a moisture-resistant device. Patients with poor eyesight or dexterity may need a device with batteries that will charge while in the unit or one that uses replaceable batteries that will last several weeks before needing to be changed. If dropping may be a problem, choose a device that is durable and will not roll when set down. Table 8.2 provides guidance for selecting the appropriate artificial larynx for a patient.

The presence of a responsible caregiver can override some physical or mental limitations of the patient. The cost of the device as well as maintenance and repair costs should also be factors in the decision.

Neck-held electrolarynges can be converted into a tube-in-the-mouth type with an oral adapter. Many companies sell these adapters. You will need to help patients decide which type is best suited for them. Table 8.3 lists manufacturers of the different types of artificial larynx devices.

Tracheoesophageal Puncture

The TEP technique is a method of voice restoration after total laryngectomy. A puncture is made through the back wall of the trachea into the esophagus, which allows air to be shunted from the trachea into the esophagus, usually creating fluent conversational speech. A valved tube is worn in the puncture opening at all times to prevent it from closing and to eliminate aspiration from

TABLE 8.2. Guidelines for selecting an artificial larynx

Types of artificial larynx devices	Considerations and requirements
Neck-held device	Absence of thick or irregular scar tissue
	An average or long neck (a short or fat neck will cause the device to press against the jaw bones or skull)
	Throat tissue must not be hardened by radiation therapy
	Absence of skin irritation or breakdown in the neck area
	Good hand control or coordination
	Good body scheme proprioception
Tube-in-the-mouth	Absence of thick or copious saliva or exceptionally acidic saliva
	Absence of tongue muscle damage or other articulation problems
	Absence of alcoholism
Pneumatic intra-oral Palate device	Good use of both hands
	Enough hand and finger dexterity to operate a wireless remote switch, remove and reinsert the device, and change a small battery
	Appropriate for patients experiencing neck pain

leaking during the swallow. The valve is removed periodically for cleaning.

The therapist should receive formal training before attempting this procedure. Table 8.4 lists potential problems with the TEP procedure and their solutions.

TABLE 8.3. Types of artificial larynxes and their manufacturers

Unit name	Type	Manufacturer or primary distributor
Artificial Larynx DSP8 and DSP81	Stoma fitted, pneumatically powered	Memacon Pres. Kennedylaan 263 P.O. Box 56 6880 AB Velp The Netherlands (85) 618708
Bruce	Neck-type, battery powered	Bruce Medical Supply 411 Waverly Oaks Rd. Waltham, MA 02254 (800) 225-8446 Fax: (617) 894-9519
Cooper-Rand Electronic Larynx	Tube-in-the-mouth, battery powered	Luminaud 8688 Tyler Blvd. Mentor, OH 44060 (216) 255-9082 (800) 255-3408
Denrick 2	Neck-type, battery powered	Luminaud 8688 Tyler Blvd. Mentor, OH 44060 (216) 255-9082 (800) 255-3408
Griffin	Neck-type, battery powered	Lauder Enterprises 11115 Whisper Hollow San Antonio, TX 78230-3609 (800) 388-8642 Fax: (210) 492-0864
Jedcom	Neck-type, battery powered	Bruce Medical Supply 411 Waverly Oaks Rd. Waltham, MA 02254 (800) 225-8446 Fax: (617) 894-9519
Nu-Vois	Neck-type, battery powered	Mountain Precision Manufacturing Co. 10688 Executive Dr. Boise, ID 83713

TABLE 8.3. (continued)

Unit name	Type	Manufacturer or primary distributor
Romet	Neck-type, battery powered	(208) 322-1111 (800) 688-6471 Romet, Inc. 9925 Mahogany Grove Ln. Las Vegas, NV 89117 (702) 233-3975
Servox	Neck-type, battery powered	Siemens Hearing Instruments, Inc. 16 East Piper Lane Suite 128 Prospect Heights, IL 60070 (800) 333-9083
SPKR	Neck-type, battery powered	Uni Manufacturers P.O. Box 607 Ontario, OR 97914 Fax: (541) 889-6567 or Dean Rosecrans P.O. Box 128 Nampa, IN 83653-0128 (800) 237-3699
Tokyo Artificial Larynx	Handheld, pneumatically powered	Artificial Speech Aids Westridge Acres 3002-8-12th St. Harlan, IA 51537 (712) 255-2389
Tru-Tone	Neck-type, battery powered	Lauder Enterprises 11115 Whisper Hollow San Antonio, TX 78230-3609 (800) 388-8642 Fax: (210) 492-0864
Ultra Voice	Palatal prosthesis	Ultra Voice 19 E Central Ave. Paoli, PA 19301 (800) 721-4848

TABLE 8.4. Tracheoesophageal puncture problems and solutions

Observed problem	Potential cause	Solution
Microstoma	Stenosis	Silicone tracheostoma vent
		Surgical revision of tracheostoma (enlargement) of the stoma
Macrostoma	Natural trachea size and tracheomalacia	Surgical revision of tracheostoma (reduction)
Leakage through prosthesis	Duckbill tip contact against posterior esophageal wall	Replace with low pressure type prosthesis
	Valve deterioration	Replace prosthesis
	Candida deposits on or in valve mechanism	Nystatin Oral Suspension swish and swallow 1 tsp bid
Leakage around prosthesis	Prosthesis is too long resulting in piston movement or track dilation	Resize to a shorter prosthesis
	Insufficient tracheoesophageal party wall thickness	Reconstruct tracheoesophageal party wall with muscle flap
	Irradiated tissue	Flap reconstruction
Granulation tissue formation	Irritation, inflammation, or tissue thickness (circumferential "doughnut" associated with presence of foreign body)	Surgical removal of tissue (circumferential "doughnut")
		Increase frequency of prosthesis removal and disinfection
Immediate post-fitting aphonia/dysphonia	Prosthesis' valved tip is stuck secondary to increased saliva viscosity	Remove prosthesis and inspect valve. Lubricate valve mechanism with vegetable oil (cooking oil)

TABLE 8.4. (continued)

Observed problem	Potential pause	Solution
Immediate post-fitting aphonia/dysphonia	Forceful stoma occlusion	Lighter finger contact when occluding the stoma
	Pharyngeal constrictor spasm	Assess voice without prosthesis*
		Transtracheal insufflation via 18 French catheter*
		Insufflation under fluoroscopy*
		Pharyngeal plexus nerve block*
Delayed post-fitting aphonia/dysphonia	Prosthesis' valved tip is stuck	Remove prosthesis and inspect valve. Lubricate valve mechanism with vegetable oil (cooking oil)
	Puncture tract closure secondary to inadequate prosthesis length	Dilate and reinsert longer prosthesis
	Failure to fully insert prosthesis	Dilate and reinsert prosthesis
Insufficient tracheostoma valve tape seal duration	Excessive system back pressure	Assess pressure during connected speech with pressure meter
		Alter prosthesis type and diameter
		Reduce speech loudness
	Failure to cleanse skin prior to valve placement	Clean skin with alcohol
		Cleanse adhesive solvent from skin surface with alcohol
	Failure to allow adhesive to dry	Wait 3–4 min before applying tape

Observed problem	Potential cause	Solution
		housing to adhesive coated skin
	Careless application or use	Reinstruct in method of application
		Remove valve prior to coughing
		Eliminate excess mucus accumulation at stoma

*Pharyngeal constrictor myotomy may be required if fluent voicing cannot be achieved.
Source: Reprinted with permission from ED Blom, RC Hamaker, SB Freeman. Postlaryngectomy Voice Restoration. In FE Lucente (ed), Highlights of the Instructional Courses (Vol. 7). St. Louis: Mosby-Year Book, 1994;9.

Established Guidelines for Determining Tracheoesophageal Puncture Candidates [7, 8]

- The patient must be motivated to improve his or her alaryngeal speech.
- The patient must have realistic expectations of postoperative speech results.
- The patient must be mentally and physically capable of caring for the prosthesis.
- The tracheostoma must be at least 1 cm in the greatest diameter (the size of a quarter is optimal, the size of a nickel is acceptable).
- The tracheostoma must be above the jugular notch of the manubrium.

- The patient must have a healthy tracheoesophageal common wall.
- The patient must be swallowing without difficulty.
- The patient must have fluent phonation on a transnasal catheter insufflation test.

If a secondary puncture is done, the patient should be fitted no sooner than 6 weeks after the puncture. This allows the patient to become accustomed to maintaining hygiene as well as satisfactory maturation of the tracheostoma.

If irradiation therapy is performed, the patient should have a TEP procedure done no sooner than 6–12 weeks postradiation to allow the acute effects of the therapy to resolve.

Insufflation Testing

Before the TEP procedure, the speech-language pathologist or laryngologist can evaluate the laryngectomized patient's ability to move air through the pharyngoesophageal junction and identify the presence of a pharyngoesophageal spasm by means of a transnasal catheter insufflation test.

1. The catheter must be inserted through the nose and advanced 25 cm to ensure that it is sufficiently below the pharyngoesophageal junction. Inserting the catheter too far or not far enough may result in a false-positive or false-negative reading. The catheter may either be connected to a syringe and a manome-

ter or to a tracheostomal housing, which adheres to the skin around the peristomal area. The patient can use his or her air to create voicing [6].

2. Voice should be produced and sustained for at least 8 seconds.

3. Voice production that is choked off spasmodically indicates a pharyngoesophageal muscle spasm or constrictor muscle hypertonicity. The patient may be able to break this pattern. If not, it can require a pharyngeal constrictor myotomy or a pharyngeal plexus neurectomy, however.

4. Failure to produce voice can result from any of the following: the patient trying to inject air as he or she would for esophageal speech (have the patient hold his or her mouth open during the test to prevent this); the patient swallowing during the test, thus preventing the air from flowing; the patient pressing too hard with his or her finger against the stoma; the catheter not being anchored properly; or air being forced into the stomach (the patient can become distended due to trapped air, indicating a pharyngoesophageal spasm).

Myotomies and Neurectomies

When a patient fails to achieve voicing during an insufflation test but desires to proceed with TEP voice restoration, one of two clinical procedures will likely be necessary to eliminate the pharyngoesophageal spasm: pharyngeal constrictor myotomy or pharyngeal plexus neurectomy. Before proceeding with these procedures, the potential for airflow after relaxation of the pharyngeal constrictor muscle can be determined by an ear, nose, and throat specialist performing a pharyngeal plexus nerve block using lidocaine or procaine (Novocain). If the patient still cannot produce voice after the block is done, a myotomy will not work.

I. Pharyngeal constrictor myotomy (cricopharyngeal myotomy)
   A. Definition: This procedure is a surgical dissection of the cricopharyngeal muscle to relax the upper esophageal sphincter.
   B. Advantage: It reduces muscle spasm and allows patient to produce TE speech.
   C. Disadvantage: It results in a lower-pitched voice, which has been judged by listeners to be of an inferior quality.
II. Pharyngeal plexus neurectomy
   A. Definition: This technique alters the tonicity of the pharynx without myotomy by modification of the motor innervation of the pharynx.
   B. Advantages:
      1. It is less anatomically destructive.
      2. It results in better sound quality speech.
      3. The procedure preserves the vascular integrity of the pharyngeal wall.
      4. It can be done during the primary laryngectomy.
      5. The technique has a low failure rate.

C. Disadvantages: It results in an incomplete neurectomy if one of the nerve branches is missed.

Note: Patients who cannot have a myotomy due to multiple radiation treatments may benefit from a botulinum neurotoxin A (Botox) injection into the pharyngeal musculature. Another alternative procedure is a mechanical hypopharyngeal dilation [6].

Procedure for Tracheoesophageal Puncture Voice Restoration

1. **Use universal precautions during the entire procedure.**
2. To prevent aspiration, instruct the patient not to swallow after the catheter is removed.
3. Check the integrity of the puncture while nothing is in it. The patient should be able to voice as well with the prosthesis out as he or she does with it in.
4. Immediately after the speech attempt, replace the catheter or use a TEP dilator.
5. If a secondary puncture patient has passed all the insufflation tests and produced sound without the prosthesis, but still has difficulty producing sound at first with the prosthesis in, it may not be due to an improper fit, but rather to lazy abdominal muscles and the poor coordination of breathing with speaking.
6. Select the type of prosthesis (duckbill versus low-pressure). Insert the prosthesis.

7. Ask the patient to attempt voicing again, and then secure the retention strap to the neck with tape.

8. Train the patient to occlude the stoma with the thumb of the nondominant hand. The patient should take a deep breath, exhale, open his or her mouth to say "ah," and occlude the stoma with as little pressure as needed. The clinician may want to occlude the stoma for the patient on the first few trials.

9. Discuss precautions, including (1) to prevent aspiration and to keep the puncture from closing, keep the tract open at all times with either a prosthesis or a dilator; (2) use an introducer to prevent aspiration of the prosthesis during insertion; (3) use good hygiene when handling the stoma and cleaning the prosthesis.

10. Monitor the patient periodically on the day of the fitting to ensure a proper fitting.

11. Bring the patient back the second day and instruct him or her on how to insert, remove, and clean the prosthesis.

12. If necessary, downsize the prosthesis several times after the initial fitting as the swelling goes down.

13. Decide if the patient can benefit from a valve or a humidifilter.

Methods of Teaching Esophageal Speech

When teaching esophageal speech, be sensitive to the fact that patients may be uncomfortable in creating a belch-like sound. After all, such behavior is discouraged in polite society. Refrain from referring to esophageal speech as burping. Rather, refer to it by its proper name, *esophageal speech*, and to the method as *air injection*.

Before beginning esophageal speech training, perform an insufflation test on the patient to see if he or she is physically capable of producing an esophageal sound. This simple procedure can save many hours of futile effort. If the insufflation test is unsuccessful, the patient may need to undergo a myotomy or a neurectomy to decrease the muscle tension in the cricopharyngeal constrictor muscle to allow development of esophageal sound.

It is also important to evaluate the patient's hearing. A hearing deficiency makes learning esophageal speech very difficult.

After the preliminary insufflation test is completed and the patient has shown an ability to create esophageal sound, the patient should be given a good description of his or her anatomy (see Figures 8.1 and 8.2) and how esophageal speech works. Explain to the patient that the amount of air required to form a new voice is the amount of air that can be trapped in the cheeks. Have the patient puff his or her cheeks to demonstrate the buildup of air pressure. Also explain that there are some sounds in the English language that can still be produced without a larynx. Have the patient say the /t/, /s/, /p/, /k/, /tʃ/, and /f/ sounds. These voiceless sounds can be used to help trap air in the upper esophagus and produce esophageal sound.

It is also a good idea to have a tape recording of someone using esophageal speech if you, the clinician, are unable to inject air yourself. It helps the patient to have something to model. Knowing that other people have accomplished this method of speaking also improves the patient's morale.

Instruct the patient to practice several hours each day. The more esophageal sound is produced, the easier it becomes. The production of the sound helps keep the throat relaxed.

During therapy sessions, it can be helpful to have the patient drink a carbonated beverage or water. A patient's mouth and throat can become very dry during a session. Learning esophageal speech is hard work!

Be aware that after several minutes of attempting to inject air, the patient may begin to feel uncomfortably bloated. This is the result of air being forced into the stomach. Encourage a real belch to relieve this pressure. Have the patient try to talk on this air. Why waste it?

Consonant Injection (The Most Efficient Method of Air Injection) [9, 10]

- Have the patient exaggerate tongue and mouth movements while saying words beginning with voiceless consonants, such as "tic-tac-toe," "puh-puh-puh," "church," "scratch," and "scotch."
- The patient should say the words slowly. The tongue pressing on the hard palate creates enough pressure to pump the air into the esophagus.
- Have the patient repeat any word that has been produced successfully over and over until the esophageal voice occurs each time.

- Next, have the patient extend the vowel sound in the words on which there is success. Some people call this "gargling" the sound.
- Once the patient is able to produce voiceless consonant words, introduce words with voiced consonants.

Glossopharyngeal Press [9, 10]

- Have the patient press the tongue against the roof of the mouth with his or her mouth closed.
- Have the patient try to force the air into the upper esophagus, using a tongue-pumping action.
- Call attention to a "klunk" sound as the air enters the esophagus. Have the patient then open the mouth to release the air and create a belch-like sound.
- Once the patient is able to create this sound, practice it over and over until it can be produced each time.
- Have the patient try to extend the sound while saying "ah." The goal is for the patient to be able to produce the sound for 1–2 seconds.
- Suggest that the patient exaggerate the movements of the mouth and tongue to help create a more intelligible speech.

Inhalation Method [9, 10]

- Have the patient take a quick, short sniff of air through the mouth.

- Have the patient attempt to say syllables or words beginning with voiceless consonants (e.g., /pah/, /tah/, /kah/).
- Have the patient take a rapid intake of air before each word.
- Practice any words produced successfully over and over.

Swallowing Method [9, 10]

- Have the patient open and close the mouth, trapping air inside.
- Have the patient press his or her lips together firmly and press the tongue firmly against the roof of the mouth and feel a small bubble of air between the tongue and the roof of the mouth.
- Next have the patient attempt to swallow this bubble of air.
- Have the patient listen for the "klunk" as the air enters the esophagus.
- After the patient hears the "klunk," tell the patient to release the sound immediately.
- Have the patient attempt to say the syllables that begin with tongue-tip alveolar consonants (e.g., "tay," "day," "toe," "doe").
- Have the patient repeat any syllable produced successfully over and over.
- Work on extending the vowel sounds of the syllables that the patient produces with ease.

REFERENCES

1. Loeb S (ed). Nursing TimeSavers: Respiratory Disorders. Springhouse, PA: Springhouse, 1994;293.
2. American Joint Committee on Cancer. AJCC Manual for Staging of Cancer (4th ed). Philadelphia: Lippincott-Raven, 1992;39.
3. Logemann JA. Evaluation and Treatment of Swallowing Disorders. San Diego: College-Hill Press, 1983;159.
4. Meyerhoff WL, Rice DH. Otolaryngology—Head and Neck Surgery. Philadelphia: Saunders, 1992.
5. Logemann JA, et al. Mechanisms of Recovery of Swallow After Supraglottic Laryngectomy. J Speech Hear Res 1994;37:965.
6. Andrews ML. Manual of Voice Treatment: Pediatrics Through Geriatrics. San Diego: Singular, 1995;309.
7. Singer MI, Blom ED, Hamaker RC. Voice Rehabilitation Following Laryngectomy. In EN Myers, JY Suen (eds), Cancer of the Head and Neck (2nd ed). New York: Churchill Livingstone, 1989;593.
8. Case JL. Clinical Management of Voice Disorders (2nd ed). Austin, TX: PRO-ED, 1991;260.
9. Lauder E. Self-Help for the Laryngectomee. San Antonio: Lauder Enterprises, 1979;24.
10. Prater RJ, Swift RW. Manual of Voice Therapy. Austin, TX: PRO-ED, 1984;267.

SUGGESTED READING

Blom ED, Hamaker RC, Freeman SB. Postlaryngectomy Voice Restoration. In FE Lucente (ed), Highlights of the Instructional Courses (Vol. 7). St. Louis: Mosby-Year Book, 1994;3.

9

Voice Disorders

Voice disorders are usually classified by either their etiology, which refers to either the cause or theory explaining the signs and symptoms, or by their perceptual characteristics, which refers to quality, pitch, loudness, and flexibility. The etiologic classification can be further divided into voice disorders of an organic origin (e.g., congenital disorders, endocrine disorders, trauma, inflammation, tumors, and neurologic disease) or voice disorders of a psychogenic origin (i.e., those resulting from emotional stress and musculoskeletal tension or psychoneurosis).

TYPES OF VOICE DISORDERS AND THEIR CHARACTERISTICS

Voice Disorders with Congenital Etiologies

Congenital Laryngeal Cysts

Congenital laryngeal cysts are small fluid-filled sacs found in the larynx that can cause swelling of the false vocal folds, aryepiglottic folds, or arytenoids.

Characteristics
- Weak or aphonic voice or cry
- Hoarseness
- Inspiratory stridor

Therapeutic Interventions
- Medicosurgical procedures to remove the cysts
- Voice therapy for persistent postsurgical hoarseness

Congenital Laryngeal Web

Congenital laryngeal web is caused by webbing of the connective tissue in the subglottic, glottic, and supraglottic regions. It is usually located at the anterior commissure and grows posteriorly.

Characteristics
- Abnormal speaking voice and cry (ranges from hoarseness to aphonia)
- Inhalatory stridor may be present

Therapeutic Interventions
- Medicosurgical procedures to dilate or remove the webbing
- Voice therapy for post surgical breathiness and hoarseness

Congenital Laryngocele

Congenital laryngocele is an air- or fluid-filled dilation or herniation of the space between the false and true vocal folds.

Characteristics
- Hoarse voice or cry

- Inspiratory stridor
- Dysphagia
- External bulge in the neck

Therapeutic Interventions

- Medicosurgical procedures
- Speech therapy not indicated

Congenital Subglottic Hemangiomas

Congenital subglottic hemangiomas are large, sessile masses usually found in the subglottic space between the true vocal folds and the lower edge of the cricoid cartilage.

Characteristics

- Inspiratory stridor
- Dyspnea and cyanosis in more severe cases
- Hoarseness
- Excessive coughing
- Dysphagia
- Cutaneous hemangiomas in 50% of patients

Therapeutic Interventions

- Medicosurgical procedures
- Speech therapy if hoarseness persists

Congenital Subglottic Stenosis

Congenital subglottic stenosis is characterized by a narrowing of the airway between the glottis and the first tracheal ring.

Characteristics

- Stridorous voice from birth
- Normal voice during crying (usually)
- Inhalatory and exhalatory stridor in severe cases

Therapeutic Interventions

- Medicosurgical procedures
- Speech therapy not indicated

Cri du Chat Syndrome

Cri du chat syndrome is caused by partial deletion of chromosome 5. The appearance of the larynx is identical to that found in laryngomalacia.

Characteristics

- Distinctive, high-pitched wail similar to the cry of a cat
- Abnormal laryngeal development
- Micrognathia
- Beak-like profile
- Microcephaly
- Hypotonia
- Hypertelorism
- Downward-slanting eyes
- Mental retardation
- Low-set ears
- Strabismus
- Midline oral clefts
- Failure to thrive
- Language and articulation delays

Therapeutic Interventions

- Speech therapy to treat cognitive and language deficits
- Articulation therapy
- Voice therapy to reduce habitually high pitch

Laryngeal Cleft

A laryngeal cleft is a vertical opening between the larynx and the esophagus. It may involve only the larynx or form a complete laryngotracheoesophageal cleft.

Characteristics

- Weak, feeble, or aphonic cry
- Feeding difficulties
- Respiration obstruction
- Repeated pneumonia

Therapeutic Interventions

- Medicosurgical procedures to close the cleft
- Voice therapy if there is structural inadequacy of the laryngeal mechanism for phonation after surgical repair

Laryngomalacia

Laryngomalacia is characterized by excessive flaccidity of the supraglottic larynx due to insufficient or delayed calcium deposition in infants. The patient will have an omega-shaped epiglottis that collapses over the glottis during inspiration. The aryepiglottic folds are close to each other and are sucked into the glottis on inspiration and blown out on exhalation.

Characteristics

- Stridor
- Voice may sound normal on exhalation, during crying, and during other types of phonation
- Low-pitched vibratory fluttering or high-pitched crowing on inhalation
- Low and narrow epiglottis with curled edges
- Approximated aryepiglottic folds
- Redundant mucosa over the arytenoid cartilages
- Dyspnea or cyanosis

Therapeutic Interventions

- Medicosurgical procedures
- Speech therapy usually not indicated

Papilloma

Papilloma is a wart-like growth that occurs in the larynx and tracheobronchial tree. The etiology is viral. The lesions are sessile or pedunculated. They arise from the anterior part of the larynx and may spread to the supraglottic region and subglottic region, and even into the trachea and bronchi. If untreated, they can produce asphyxiation and death [1].

Characteristics

- Usually occurs between the ages of 2 and 4 years
- Usually disappears during puberty, but may persist into or arise during adulthood

- Voice quality ranges from hoarseness to aphonia depending on the size of the lesion
- Possible croupy cough
- Possible wheezing stridor on inhalation and exhalation
- Dyspnea

Therapeutic Interventions

- Medicosurgical procedures
- Speech therapy if hoarseness persists after surgical removal of papilloma

Voice Disorders Associated with Laryngeal Trauma

Burns to the Larynx

Burns to the larynx are usually caused by inhalation of hot air or gases, the ingestion of hot foods or liquids, or by ingestion of corrosive chemicals.

Characteristics

- Hoarse and breathy to aphonia
- Painful phonation
- Possible stridor and respiratory obstruction
- Infection
- Ulceration followed by granulated and fibrotic lesions in chemical burns

Therapeutic Interventions

- Vocal rest program
- Direct voice therapy techniques contraindicated

Contact Ulcer (Musculoskeletal Tension)

A contact ulcer is usually a bilateral sessile benign lesion on the vocal process of each arytenoid cartilage resulting from vocal abuse.

Characteristics

- Complaint of laryngeal pain
- Vocal fatigue
- Referred pain to lateral neck or ear, especially during swallowing
- Nonproductive cough
- Hoarse, breathy, low-pitched voice
- Complaints of a lump or tickling sensation in the throat

Therapeutic Interventions

- Education in vocal hygiene
- Vocal rest program
- Elimination of vocal abuse patterns
- Training in optimal pitch
- Stress management and stress reduction strategies
- Biofeedback

Keratosis of the Larynx

Keratosis of the larynx refers to laryngeal lesions characterized by abnormal growth and/or maturation of the epithelium.

Hyperkeratosis

Hyperkeratosis is a benign, plaque-like, irregular thickening of the laryngeal mucosa characterized by abnormal growth and/or maturation of the epithelium that results from laryngeal trauma, smoking, vocal misuse and abuse, chronic laryngitis, alcohol abuse, or radiation injury.

Characteristics

- Hoarseness
- Lowered vocal pitch

Therapeutic Interventions

- Vocal hygiene program
- Elimination of vocal abuse patterns

Leukoplakia

Laryngeal leukoplakia is characterized by premalignant white patches on the mucous membranes of the larynx resulting from chronic irritation to the larynx as in hyperkeratosis. This condition is not usually responsive to voice therapy.

Characteristics

- Hoarseness
- Patient may be asymptomatic

Therapeutic Interventions

- Removal of laryngeal irritants
- Vocal rest

Laryngitis (Inflammation)

Laryngitis is characterized by inflammatory reactions of the vocal fold and surrounding tissues caused by viruses, bacteria, trauma, smoking, or vocal misuse.

Acute Laryngitis

Acute laryngitis results from infection (voice therapy is contraindicated because the vocal symptoms will subside when the upper respiratory tract infection clears and the vocal cord edema decreases).

Chronic Acute Laryngitis

Chronic acute laryngitis is characterized by severe atrophy of the laryngeal mucosa (responds poorly to voice therapy; voice therapy is contraindicated).

Chronic Hypertrophic Laryngitis

Chronic hypertrophic laryngitis is characterized by enlargement of the laryngeal epithelium due to chronic laryngeal irritation (responds poorly to voice therapy).

Chronic Nonspecific Laryngitis

Chronic nonspecific laryngitis is characterized by long-standing inflammation of the laryngeal mucosa due to laryngeal trauma (e.g., smoking, vocal abuse, or persistent mouth breathing).

Characteristics of All Forms of Laryngitis

- Hoarse, low-pitched voice
- Dysphonia
- Vocal fatigue
- Nonproductive cough
- Sore throat
- Urge to clear the throat

Therapeutic Interventions for Chronic Nonspecific Laryngitis

- Elimination of laryngeal irritants
- Medical intervention
- Voice therapy to eliminate vocal abuse and misuse

Mechanical Trauma

Mechanical trauma is characterized by a direct injury to the laryngeal submucosal tissue, causing edema and hematoma formation or an injury that can cause intubation granuloma, traumatic laryngeal web, or dislocation or fracture of the laryngeal cartilages. Some causes of laryngeal trauma include motor vehicle accidents, gunshot wounds, knife wounds, endotracheal intubation, and indwelling nasogastric tubes.

Characteristics

- Hoarseness
- Dysphonia or aphonia
- Possible dysphagia
- Persistent cough

Therapeutic Interventions

- Vocal rest
- Medical intervention for laryngeal webbing and dislocation or fracture of the laryngeal cartilages
- Voice therapy to increase glottal tension if vocal cords are paralyzed or weakened

Vocal Nodules (Musculoskeletal Tension)

Vocal nodules are bilateral and symmetric benign extensions of epithelium at the junction of the anterior one-third and posterior two-thirds of the true vocal folds caused by vocal abuse and misuse.

Characteristics
- Hoarse, breathy vocal quality
- Low-pitched voice
- Nonproductive cough

Therapeutic Interventions
- Vocal rest program
- Elimination of vocal abuse patterns
- Education in vocal hygiene

Vocal Polyps (Musculoskeletal Tension)

Vocal polyps are benign, unilateral extensions of the epithelium on the free margin of the vocal folds usually at the junction of the anterior and middle one-third of the vocal fold margin that results from vocal fold trauma. They can be a fluid-filled or blood-engorged sessile or pedunculated mass.

Characteristics
- Diplophonia
- Sudden pitch breaks with pedunculated polyps
- Hoarse, breathy vocal quality with sessile polyps

Therapeutic Interventions
- Vocal rest program
- Elimination of vocal abuse patterns
- Education in vocal hygiene

Organic Voice Disorders Due to Neurologic Disease (see Chapters 3 and 6)

Neurologic voice disorders exhibit the same relationship between anatomic location of lesion and acoustic effect as the dysarthrias. In fact, neurologic voice disorders, technically, are dysarthrias; although they occur in isolation, most often they are embedded in a more widespread complex of respiratory, resonatory, and articulatory dysarthric signs. Dysphonia can be the first sign of neurologic disease, the remainder of the dysarthria following as the disease progresses. [1]

These dysphonias are characterized in Chapter 3 under the section on motor speech disorders, and dysarthrias.

Voice Disorders Associated with Endocrine Dysfunction

Voice disorders due to endocrine dysfunction are not amenable to voice therapy. These disorders are included, however, to help the clinician differentiate a voice disorder due to this etiology from those that do respond to treatment and to help the clinician make the proper referrals.

Amyloidosis

Laryngeal amyloidosis occurs as an atypical laryngeal nodule or subglottic stenosis. It is usually misdiagnosed as a vocal nodule or idiopathic subglottic stenosis [1].

Characteristics

- Breathy voice
- Excessively low-pitched voice
- Hoarse voice
- Atypical laryngeal nodule
- Subglottic stenosis

Therapeutic Interventions

- Hormone therapy
- Speech therapy not indicated

Hyperthyroidism

Hyperthyroidism is caused by an abnormality of the thyroid gland in which secretion of thyroid hormone is usually increased and is no longer under regulatory control of hypothalamic-pituitary centers.

Characteristics

- Breathy voice
- Reduced loudness
- Anxiety
- Irritability
- Fatigability

Therapeutic Interventions

- Hormone therapy
- Speech therapy not indicated

Hypothyroidism

Hypothyroidism is caused by insufficient secretion of thyroxin by the thyroid glands.

Characteristics

- Hoarseness, coarse or gravelly voice
- Excessively low-pitched voice
- Distortions of articulation, particularly the anterior lingual sounds
- Lethargy
- Intolerance to cold
- Puffiness around the eyes
- Dry skin
- Loss of frontal hair
- In severe cases, ataxia and ataxic dysarthria
- In severe cases, changes in intellect, language, and personality

Therapeutic Interventions

- Hormone therapy
- Speech therapy not indicated

Virilization

Virilization refers to the development of male sex characteristics in females due to excess secretion of androgenic hormones. The secretion of this hormone causes the larynx to grow to a larger-than-normal size.

Characteristics

- Abnormally low-pitched voice

- Hoarseness
- Facial hair
- Possible falsetto pitch breaks

Therapeutic Interventions

- Hormone therapy
- Speech therapy not indicated

Psychogenic Voice Disorders

Conversion Dysphonia, Conversion Aphonia, Conversion Muteness

Conversion dysphonia, conversion aphonia, and conversion muteness are characterized by total or partial loss of phonatory ability due to a psychoneurosis.

Characteristics

- Mild disruption of vocal function to complete loss of the voice
- Unaffected nonvocal acts (crying, coughing, sighing, laughing)
- History of emotional stress
- Sudden onset of symptoms
- Symptoms exaggerated if found in combination with a laryngeal pathology

Therapeutic Interventions [2]

- Counseling
- Providing patient education and a physiologic, not a psychological, explanation of the voice loss

- Having the patient produce vegetative vocal functions (e.g., coughing, clearing the throat, yawning, sighing)
- Having the patient shape the vegetative vocal sounds into a vowel sound (e.g., /a/ or /o/) until consistent
- While the patient is using the vegetative vocal sounds, having him or her attempt other vowel productions until consistent
- Having the patient attempt to produce vowels without using a vegetative sound until consistent
- Having the patient attempt to say nonsense syllables starting with /h/
- Having the patient attempt to say words beginning with vowel sounds before words beginning with consonants
- After the patient stabilizes the word level, having him or her attempt phrases and sentences
- Having the patient converse with a friend or family member

Mutational Falsetto (Puberphonia)

Mutational falsetto (puberphonia) is characterized by the failure to eliminate the higher prepubescent voice with a lower-pitched voice in postpubescence. The larynx is structurally normal.

Characteristics

- High-pitched, breathy voice
- Occasional drops in pitch level
- Larynx elevated high in the neck and tilted downward

Therapeutic Interventions [2]

- Having the patient shape vegetative vocal productions into a normal voice (e.g., coughing, grunting, or clearing the throat)
- Pointing out the lower-pitched voice to the patient as he or she coughs or clears the throat to reveal the capacity for a lower-pitched voice
- If the patient cannot produce a lower-pitched voice with a cough, having the patient gently pull the larynx lower in the neck with his or her hands while he or she coughs
- After the patient establishes a lower-pitched voice with a cough, having the patient cough and immediately say /a/; repeat until a lower voice is consistently produced
- Having the patient attempt other vowel sounds using a cough until consistent
- Having the patient eliminate the cough and produce vowels in isolation until consistent
- Having the patient attempt to produce a lower-pitched voice in syllables, words, phrases, and sentences
- Having the patient carry over the new voice into different speaking situations

Spasmodic Dysphonia

Spasmodic dysphonia may either be functional in origin, or it may have an organic basis. There are two types: adductor and abductor spasmodic dysphonia.

Abductor Spasmodic Dysphonia

Abductor spasmodic dysphonia is a severe, breathy dysphonia in which the vocal folds episodically abduct to the lateral position.

Characteristics

- Intermittent moments of aphonia and breathiness
- Impairment of voiced or voiceless phoneme distinctions
- Difficulty with the transition from voiceless consonants to a vowel in a stressed syllable
- Approximation of the vocal folds that then abruptly abduct widely on phonation

Therapeutic Interventions [1, 2]

- Having the patient voice all unvoiced consonants (e.g., "coffee cake" will become "goffee gake")
- Telling the patient to keep the vocal cords vibrating through all connected speech

Adductor Spasmodic Dysphonia

Adductor spasmodic dysphonia is a voice disorder in which the vocal folds are approximated so tightly that the patient cannot produce sustained vocal fold vibration.

Characteristics

- Nonspecific hoarseness
- Vocal catches and pitch breaks
- Laryngospasms

- Strained, squeezed, staccato phonation in advanced cases
- Usually unaffected laughing, singing, shouting, and coughing
- Difficulty breathing
- Muscle pain in the upper chest
- Facial grimaces
- Neck contractions
- Synkinetic eye blinking
- True and false vocal folds hyperadduct in intermittent and irregular spasms

Therapeutic Interventions [1, 2]

- Can be managed surgically through a recurrent laryngeal nerve resection or through the use of a botulinum toxin injection
- Using techniques that reduce laryngeal tension (e.g., chewing technique, chanting technique, and biofeedback). (These are trial therapy methods used before surgery; see Table 9.1.)

Ventricular Dysphonia

Ventricular dysphonia is a condition that develops due to excessive muscular tension in the laryngeal area or as a result of disease or paralysis of the true vocal folds in which the false vocal folds are used for phonation instead of the true vocal folds.

Characteristics

- Hoarse, low-pitched voice

TABLE 9.1. Twenty-five facilitating approaches in voice therapy

Facilitating approach	Phonatory process affected			Parameter of voice affected	
	Mass/size	Approxi-mation	Loud-ness	Pitch	Quality
1. Altering tongue position		X		X	X
2. Biofeedback	X	X	X	X	X
3. Change of loudness	X	X	X	X	
4. Chant talk		X	X		X
5. Chewing approach	X	X	X	X	X
6. Digital manipulation	X			X	
7. Ear training	X	X	X	X	X
8. Elimination of abuses	X	X	X	X	X
9. Elimination of hard glottal attack		X	X		X
10. Establish new pitch	X			X	X
11. Explanation of problem	X	X	X	X	X
12. Feedback	X	X	X	X	
13. Gargle approach		X			X
14. Hierarchy analysis	X	X	X	X	X
15. Inhalation phonation		X		X	
16. Masking	X	X	X	X	X
17. Negative practice	X	X	X	X	X
18. Open-mouth approach	X		X	X	X
19. Pitch inflections	X	X	X	X	
20. Place the voice	X	X		X	X
21. Pushing approach		X	X		X
22. Relaxation	X	X	X	X	X
23. Respiration training		X	X		X
24. Voice rest	X	X			
25. Yawn-sigh approach	X	X	X	X	X

X = the particular facilitation approach effective for that phonatory process or parameter of voice.

Source: Reprinted with permission from DR Boone. The Voice and Voice Therapy (3rd ed). Englewood Cliffs, NJ: Prentice-Hall, 1983.

- Restricted vocal range
- Reduced loudness
- Thickened false vocal folds

Therapeutic Interventions

- Providing patient education and a detailed physiologic explanation of the problem
- Having the patient practice phonation while inhaling until the phonation is consistent
- Having the patient match the pitch during inhalation phonation with the pitch during exhalation until consistent
- Having the patient phonate a vowel sound using the same pitch
- Having the patient vary pitch when there is consistent success

VOICE EVALUATION

Before beginning a voice evaluation, obtain a full report from the referring otolaryngologist. **Never** treat a voice disorder without an initial diagnosis from a medical physician. Life-threatening conditions can go undetected without the use of proper diagnostic equipment. Tape-record the session. To continue with a motor and sensory evaluation of the speech mechanism, see Chapters 3 (motor speech evaluation) and 4 (cranial nerve assessment).

Voice Evaluation Procedures*

I.   Informal introduction period: Make observations about the patient's behavior, posture, breathing, facial expressions, eye contact, and so forth.

II. Obtain a case history including the following:

    A. Biographic information (e.g., date of birth, marital status, number of children)

    B. Health history (e.g., allergies, smoker or non-smoker, accidents, operations, medications)

    C. Onset and course of the voice disorder

    D. Other symptoms (e.g., dysphagia, nasal regurgitation, aphasia, apraxia, dysarthria)

    E. History of previous therapy

    F. Patient description of the disorder and his or her rating of the severity

    G. Patient description of how the disorder affects his or her life and how others react to the disorder

    H. Patient explanation of the possible cause of the voice disorder

III. Obtain a voice sample during reading. Have the patient read a paragraph from either the Rainbow Passage (see G Fairbanks. Voice and Articulation Drillbook [2nd ed]. New York: Harper & Row, 1960, for this passage) or the Grandfather Passage

*Source: This section was adapted from RJ Prater, RW Swift. Manual of Voice Therapy. Austin, TX: PRO-ED, 1984.

(see FL Darley, AE Aronson, JR Brown. Motor Speech Disorders. Philadelphia: Saunders, 1975, for this passage). Assess the patient's performance based on the following:

A. Rate
B. Voice quality
C. Intelligibility
D. Use of respiratory system
E. Clavicular breathing
F. Thoracic breathing
G. Diaphragmatic-abdominal breathing

IV. Assess the patient's sustained vowel production. Time the production with a stopwatch. (Fifteen to 20 seconds is normal, 15 seconds minimum for adult males and 14.3 seconds minimum for adult females are normal; 10 seconds for a child is normal.)

V. Have the patient sustain /s/ and /z/. Time the production with a stopwatch. A patient should be able to sustain the /z/ for about the same length of time as the /s/. (Twenty to 25 seconds is normal for adults; 10 seconds is normal for a child with no vocal fold pathology and no respiratory difficulty.) Sustaining the /s/ 20% longer than the /z/ indicates vocal fold pathology.

VI. Evaluate the patient's vocal fold adduction (glottal closure). Instruct the patient to cough sharply, clear the throat, or produce a vowel with a hard glottal attack. Neuromuscular weakness is indicated by a "mushy" cough, weak throat clearing, or a soft glottal attack.

VII. Assess the patient's optimal pitch. Have the patient say "uh-huh." Next, have the patient yawn and sigh. The pitch produced from these two exercises should be the patient's optimal pitch. Compare this pitch with habitual pitch during the paragraph reading to determine if the patient is using the most efficient pitch. The difference in pitch should be less than two tones.

VIII. Assess the patient's pitch range. Have the patient begin to sing or count in the middle of his or her vocal range and go down one tone with each number or note until the patient reaches the lowest note in his or her range. Repeat the procedure, having the patient go up a tone until the patient reaches the highest note in his or her range. Repeat each procedure three times.

IX. Make a subjective judgment about the patient's loudness level. Too loud? Too soft? Normal?

X. Assess vocal quality by the following:

A. Breathiness (Have patient phonate different vowels while lifting himself or herself out of a chair with his or her hands.)

B. Harshness

C. Hoarseness

D. Vocal fry (Note frequency, average duration, and where it occurs in words, phrases, and sentences.)

XI. Assess hypernasality. Have the patient alternately sustain /i/ and /u/. Compress and release the patient's nostrils. If velopharyngeal closure is adequate, there should be no noticeable alteration in vowel quality as the nose is pinched. If there is poor velopharyngeal closure, a flutter-like sound is heard.

XII. Assess the patient's hyponasality. Have the patient read a word list or passage containing /m/, /n/, and /ng/. Listen for these substitutions: /b/ for /m/, /d/ for /n/, and /g/ for /ng/. Also, compress and release the nostrils as the patient reads. Listen for changes in voice quality. No change indicates hyponasality. Another method is to have the patient hum. An inability to hum clearly indicates hyponasality.

XIII. Check for cul-de-sac resonance. Have the patient phonate /a/ and observe if the tongue is retracted posteriorly. If so, have the patient read word lists containing tongue-tip sounds such as "did," "zip," "dip," "weed," "bit," "teeth," "paid," "sis," and "dizzy" to move the tongue to a forward position. Note improvement in overall vocal resonance.

XIV. Check for excessive anterior tongue carriage. Have the patient read words containing many back vowels and the back consonants /k/ and /g/ (e.g., "cook," "kook," "go," "good," and "cog"). Note any improvement in vocal resonance.

XV. Assess the patient's endurance. To assess the patient's ability to maintain sufficient muscular effort over a time period long enough to permit effective communication, have the patient count rapidly to 200. Note changes in phonation, velopharyngeal closure, or articulation.

XVI. Check for sites of vocal hypertension. Observe tension in the muscles of the face and neck, listen for a strained voice quality and hard glottal attacks. Note patient complaints of laryngeal pain.

Pathologies Associated with Perceptual Voice Characteristics*

Possible etiologies of faulty pitch
   Diplophonia
   Mutational falsetto
Possible etiologies of pitch decreases
   Large-mass lesions (e.g., polypoid degeneration, nodules, vocal fold cancer)
   Endocrine conditions (e.g., hypothyroidism, virilization, acromegaly)
   Trauma or irritation (e.g., hyperplasia, contact ulcers, granuloma, vocal fold edema, acute laryngitis)
   Psychogenic factors (e.g., chronic stress or anxiety, habitual low pitch)
Possible etiologies of pitch increases
   Pathologies and anomalies (e.g., laryngeal web, cancer of the glottis or supraglottis, sulcus vocalis)
   Endocrine conditions
   Psychogenic factors (e.g., conversion dysphonia, mutational falsetto, habitual high pitch)

*This is not an exhaustive list.

Hearing impairment

Possible etiologies of diplophonia

Vocal polyps

Unilateral paralysis of a true vocal fold (unilateral recurrent laryngeal nerve damage)

Vibration of the ventricular folds

Hyperfunctioning of the vocal mechanism

Possible etiologies for excessive noise (stridor) during inspiration or expiration

Asthma

Nasal blockage

Laryngeal neoplasm

Laryngeal webs

Abductor paresis or paralysis of vocal folds in the paramedian position

Recent decannulation resulting in edema of the laryngeal tissues

Possible etiologies for shortness of breath

Asthma

Emphysema

Chronic pulmonary disease

Possible etiologies for decreased maximum phonation time

Glottic lesions

Interarytenoidal lesions

Paralysis or paresis of the vagus nerve

Insufficient or inefficient respiratory functioning

Neurologic involvement

Faulty learned pattern of speaking

Possible etiologies of monotoned voice
  Deafness
  Depression
  Dysarthria
Possible etiologies of diminished loudness levels
  Vocal fold paralysis
  Parkinson's disease
  Bulbar paralysis
  Mass lesions of the vocal folds
  Myasthenia gravis
  Personality characteristics (e.g., shyness)
  Cultural variation
  Dysarthria
Possible etiologies for excessive loudness levels
  Poor hearing acuity
  Personality disturbance
  Neurologic disorders that cause respiratory and vocal
    fold hyperfunction (e.g., ataxic dysarthrias, hyper-
    kinetic dysarthrias)
Possible etiologies for breathiness
  Vocal folds that are bowed (bilateral damage of the
    superior laryngeal nerve)
  Paralysis of one or both of the true vocal folds in the
    abducted position
  One or both true vocal folds paralyzed in the parame-
    dian position (unilateral or bilateral damage to the
    recurrent laryngeal nerve)
  Myasthenia gravis
  Dysarthria

Mass lesions (e.g., nodules, polyps, cysts, laryngeal cancer, hematoma)

Psychogenic factors (e.g., conversion dysphonia)

Laryngeal web

Possible etiologies for harshness

Structural alterations of the larynx

Dysarthria

Poor vocal habits

Hearing impairment

Possible etiologies for hoarseness

Neurologic disease

Structural alterations of the larynx (e.g., laryngeal cancer, nodules, polyps, cysts, papilloma, leukoplakia)

Laryngeal edema (e.g., nonspecific laryngitis)

Dysarthria

Possible etiologies for hypernasality

Clefts of the hard and/or soft palate

Submucous clefts

Inadequate velar length

Unusually deep pharynx

Injury or trauma causing paralysis or paresis of the velum

Dysarthria

Paralysis or paresis of the pharyngeal constrictor muscles

Myasthenia gravis

Muscular dystrophy

Poliomyelitis

Surgical removal of tonsils and adenoids
Conversion reaction
Deafness
Possible etiologies for hyponasality
Deviated septum
Nasal polyps
Enlarged adenoids
Improper velar timing
Edema of nasal membranes
Nasal papilloma
Tumors
Mucosal congestion (e.g., allergic rhinitis and acute
rhinitis)
High palatal arch
Foreign objects in the nasal cavity (e.g., crayons, but-
tons, or beans)
Postsurgical repair
Nasal deformity
Patulous eustachian tube

REFERENCES

1. Aronson AE. Clinical Voice Disorders (3rd ed). New York: Thieme,
   1990;57,193.
2. Prater RJ, Swift RW. Manual of Voice Therapy. Austin, TX: PRO-
   ED, 1984;25.

SUGGESTED READING

Andrews ML. Manual of Voice Treatment: Pediatrics Through Geriatrics.
   San Diego: Singular, 1995.

Boone DR. The Voice and Voice Therapy (3rd ed). Englewood Cliffs, NJ: Prentice-Hall, 1983.

Case JL. Clinical Management of Voice Disorders (2nd ed). Austin, TX: PRO-ED, 1991.

Darley FL, Aronson AE, Brown JR. Motor Speech Disorders. Philadelphia: Saunders, 1975.

Fairbanks G. Voice and Articulation Drillbook (2nd ed). New York: Harper & Row, 1960.

Morrison M, Rammage L. The Management of Voice Disorders. San Diego: Singular, 1994.

10

Management of Ventilator Patients

Research has shown that patients who have had prolonged intubation may be at increased risk for aspiration after extubation or tracheostomy. The presence of a gag and cough reflex is thought to protect against aspiration in this population, but the presence of these reflexes correlates poorly with the incidence of aspiration. Aspiration may occur despite an inflated endotracheal (ET) cuff balloon in patients with either an oral ET tube or a tracheostomy tube. Even though the patients may have no evidence of any central or peripheral neurologic dysfunction, the swallowing dysfunction may persist after the tracheostomy tube is removed.

The cause of swallowing dysfunction is still unclear. It is now believed, however, that the defects may be secondary to muscle atrophy, dyscoordination, or diminished proprioception rather than motor nerve injury [1]. Several authors report specific problems related to the presence of tracheostomy tubes:

- Prolonged orotracheal intubation with or without tracheostomy tubes may cause prolonged and severe swallowing dysfunction [1].
- Inflated tracheostomy cuffs restrict the upward laryngeal movement that protects the airway [2].
- The esophagus may become compressed by the tube's pushing posteriorly on the common wall between the trachea and the esophagus [2].
- Swallowing dysfunction may persist after the tracheostomy tube is removed [1].

It is very important to note that bedside tests do not adequately assess for aspiration in these patients. A large percentage of these patients may have a normal examination and still be aspirating.

The most common swallowing defects found in tracheostomy- and ventilator-dependent patients during fluoroscopic testing are the following:

- A delayed triggering of the swallowing response
- Decreased pharyngeal peristalsis (pharyngeal pooling)
- Inconsistent triggering of the swallowing reflex
- Suppression of the cough reflex

CHART REVIEW

A bedside evaluation should begin with a careful review of the patient's medical history. Information should be gathered from the patient's chart, the physician, nursing staff, respiratory therapist, family members, and the patient. In the review of the chart of a ventilator-dependent patient, the following information can be valuable in determining the possible etiology of the dysphagia and methods of treatment:

- Admitting diagnosis
- Cause of the respiratory failure (e.g., myocardial infarction, pneumonia, lung cancer, chronic obstructive pulmonary disease)
- Length of time the patient has been tracheostomized or on a ventilator
- Ventilator rate (e.g., continuous positive airway pressure [CPAP], positive end-expiratory pressure [PEEP], controlled mode ventilation)
- Whether the patient currently has pneumonia
- A history of cerebrovascular accident (CVA), Alzheimer's disease, or anoxia
- A history of coronary artery bypass graft surgery
- Dysphagia complaints and symptoms
- A history of apnea
- Whether the patient is under diet orders or is fed by a nasogastric (NG) or percutaneous endoscopic gastrostomy (PEG) tube
- Results of any chest x-ray reports
- Results of any computer-assisted tomography scan or magnetic resonance imaging tests
- Medications that suppress cognitive function or any psychoactive drugs (e.g., phenytoin [Dilantin], carbamazepine [Tegretol], amitriptyline [Elavil], fluoxe-

tine [Prozac], chlorpromazine [Thorazine], thioridazine [Mellaril], prochlorperazine [Compazine], haloperidol decanoate [Haldol] (Such drugs can impair swallowing, especially if there is an underlying swallowing dysfunction [3].)

- Results of any pulmonary tests to determine if the patient can tolerate any amount of aspiration
- Whether the patient is currently receiving respiratory treatments and how frequently
- The presence of infectious conditions such as methicillin-resistant *Staphylococcus aureus*
- The presence of fever or temperature spikes
- Type and size of tracheostomy tube and whether the inner and outer cannulas are fenestrated
- If the patient is off the ventilator for any time during the day
- Frequency of suctioning
- Whether the cuff can be deflated and how long the patient can tolerate the cuff being deflated
- Whether there is a history of anatomic abnormalities (e.g., fistulas, granulomas, stenosis) related to intubation or tracheostomy

A glossary is provided at the end of this book to help the clinician in interpreting the ventilator terminology found during the chart review.

Keep in mind the following:

- Silent aspirators tend to be older than 60 years [4].

- Silent aspirators are more likely to have expressive aphasia [4].
- Aspirators are more likely to have brain stem or multi-lobe involvement [4].
- Brain stem CVAs exhibit reduced laryngeal closure [5].
- A patient with a recent CVA has a higher potential for aspiration [4].

BEDSIDE EVALUATION OF VENTILATOR-DEPENDENT PATIENTS

Before a ventilator-dependent patient is given any bolus, a thorough preliminary bedside assessment should take place.

1. Examine the oral anatomy and check for oral motor control.
2. Check the abundance and viscosity of the patient's secretions. If the patient has excess secretions, he or she will need to be suctioned orally and through the tracheostomy tube.
3. Check for the presence of a cuff, the type of cuff, and whether it is inflated or deflated.
4. **Always check with the doctor or respiratory nurse to see if the patient can tolerate having the cuff deflated.**
5. Check for the presence of a fenestrated tracheostomy tube. A fenestrated inner cannula is another potential source of entry of food and secretions.
6. Assess the patient's gag reflex, voluntary and reflexive cough, vocal quality, and volitional swallow.
7. Check the skin color and condition.

8. Check the patient's pulse rate (the normal rate is 60–80 beats per minute).

9. Check the patient's respiratory quality during inspiration and expiration.

10. Assess the patient's cognitive status. Is the patient stuporous or alert? Can he or she follow commands? Impaired cognition can cause swallowing dysfunction at either the oral or pharyngeal level. It can manifest itself as impaired oral strength and coordination, delayed and inconsistent triggering of the swallow response, suppressions of the gag and cough reflex, and increased risk of aspiration.

11. Check for the presence of an NG tube or PEG tube. Large NG tubes have been found to prevent complete epiglottic closure, placing the patient at even further risk for aspiration [6].

Oral intake should be deferred until at least partial cuff deflation is achieved. An individual who is so medically fragile as to preclude cuff deflation is usually not a candidate for significant oral intake [7].

To begin assessing the swallow of a ventilator dependent patient with an inflated cuff, do the following:*

1. Ask for medical clearance before deflating a cuff. If the patient has a speaking valve, it may be worn during

---

*A negative evaluation—one in which there are no signs of aspiration—**does not absolutely rule out aspiration.** Further clinical studies are needed to prove aspiration is not present. A positive evaluation—one in which there are signs of aspiration—prevents an unnecessary videofluoroscopic study.

the bedside evaluation to normalize pharyngeal pressures.

2. **Use universal precautions.**

3. Have the nurse suction the oropharyngeal cavity to prevent any pooled secretions from descending into the trachea after the cuff is deflated.

4. Deflate the cuff either partially or fully by inserting a 5- or 10-ml syringe into the cuff pilot balloon and withdraw the air from the cuff very slowly. Leave the syringe attached to the tubing for later reinflation of the cuff. Slow deflation allows positive lung pressure to push secretions upward from the bronchi. Cuff deflation may also stimulate a cough reflex, producing additional secretions.

5. Have the patient dry swallow. Look and feel for laryngeal elevation.

6. Listen to the patient's voice quality for any wet or gurgling sounds.

7. Ask the patient to swallow either water or ice chips with blue food coloring added. The blue dye will allow you to see if aspiration has occurred.

8. Recheck the patient's voice quality.

9. Have the nurse suction through the tracheostomy tube for signs of aspiration.

10. Discontinue the evaluation if the patient has signs of aspiration around the tracheostomy site or with suctioning.

11. If there are no signs of aspiration, repeat steps 7 through 9 for several swallows. Allow breaks as needed. Have the nurse suction after each swallow.

12. Try various food consistencies on following days, using only one consistency each day so that you will be able to tell which consistency is aspirated.

13. Reinflate the cuff after the test is concluded. Check for a leak-free cuff seal. Even with minimal cuff inflation, no air should be felt coming from the patient's mouth, nose, or tracheostomy site. The patient should not be able to speak.

14. Ask the nursing staff to monitor the patient for signs of aspiration in subsequent suctionings for the next 24 hours.

To evaluate tracheostomy collar patients who have inflated cuffs, do the following:

1.   Always ask for medical clearance before deflating a cuff.

2.   **Use universal precautions.**

3.   Have the nurse suction the patient's oropharyngeal cavity to prevent any pooled secretions from descending into the trachea after the cuff is deflated.

4.   Deflate the cuff either partially or fully by inserting a 5- or 10-ml syringe into the cuff pilot balloon and very slowly withdrawing the air from the cuff. Leave the syringe attached to the tubing for later reinflation of the cuff.

5.   Occlude the tracheostomy tube and have the patient dry swallow. Look and feel for laryngeal elevation.

6.   Have the nurse suction orally and through the patient's tracheostomy tube to remove excess secretions.

7.   Listen to the patient's voice quality for any wet or gurgling sounds.

8.   Ask the patient to swallow either water or ice chips with blue food coloring added.

9.   Have the patient phonate while you occlude the tracheostomy tube.

10.   Listen for any wetness in the patient's voice. Have the patient cough or clear his or her throat.

11.   After the vocalization, ask the patient to pant for several seconds. This will cause any material pooling in the pharynx to be shaken loose and fall into the airway.

12.   After having the patient pant, have him or her vocalize again.

13.   Give the patient another bolus. Occlude the tracheostomy tube during exhalation and swallowing to facilitate pressures that drive the bolus through the pharynx.

14.   After each swallow have the nurse suction the patient through the tracheostomy tube to check for signs of aspiration. Allow breaks as needed.

15.   Discontinue the evaluation if there are signs of aspiration around the tracheostomy site or with suctioning.

16.   If no aspiration is evident, you will still need to request a videofluoroscopic examination, since a bedside blue-dye test is inconclusive.

17. Try various food consistencies on following days using only one consistency each day to tell which consistency is aspirated.

18. Reinflate the cuff after the test is concluded. Check for a leak-free cuff seal. Even with minimal cuff inflation, no air should be felt coming from the patient's mouth, nose, or tracheostomy site. The patient should not be able to speak.

19. Ask the nursing staff to monitor the patient for signs of aspiration in subsequent suctionings for the next 24 hours.

It should be noted that occasionally a cuffed tracheostomy tube will not completely occlude the trachea because of tracheal wall deviations or misfit tubes. Therefore, aspiration can occur around the cuffed tube. If a patient has food sitting on top of the cuff, the food will eventually ooze around the cuff and be aspirated [8].

If a videofluoroscopic test is not possible immediately and the doctor insists on feeding the patient without one, put the patient on 24-hour blue-dye monitoring and monitor for any temperature spikes in the next 24–48 hours.

Aspiration can also be detected through the use of glucose oxidase test strips. These strips can be used to measure the amount of glucose in tracheal secretions. This method is more sensitive in detecting aspiration than the visualization of blue dye in tracheal secretions after suctioning.

POSSIBLE SUCTIONING COMPLICATIONS

Bedside swallowing evaluations typically require frequent suctioning. This suctioning can result in the following complications:

- Tissue trauma to the pharyngeal and endobronchial mucosa causing bleeding
- Pneumonia caused by suction catheters introducing bacteria into the patient
- Coughing (Excessive coughing during suctioning can be extremely tiring, painful, and traumatic. There is a possibility that coughing will fracture ribs as well as cause severe fatigue and extreme soreness. Excessive coughing could also cause the patient to vomit.)
- Hypoxemia (Hypoxemia is a serious concern because suctioning evacuates large amounts of gas from the airway along with the secretions. If hypoxemia is a concern, have the ventilator supply 100% oxygen for 1 minute before suctioning.)

VIDEOFLUOROSCOPIC TESTING

Many tracheostomized and ventilator-dependent patients are able to undergo a videofluoroscopic test. Candidates for this procedure include the following:

- Patients who are able to remain alert for at least an hour
- Patients who are medically stable and can tolerate being transported

- Patients who can follow instructions and participate
- Optimally, patients who can tolerate either partial or full cuff deflation

During the videofluoroscopic testing, have the patient swallow with and without finger occlusion of the tracheostomy tube. Occlusion of the tracheostomy tube can be used to restore expiratory air flow, permitting the patient to use an effective cough, throat clear, or other techniques that necessitate the accumulation of subglottic air pressure [7]. Placement of a speaking valve during testing can increase the patient's ability to obtain subglottic pressure and increase the potential for clearance of any material remaining in the pharynx. Also, check with the doctor to see if the NG tube can be removed during testing.

1. Ask for medical clearance before deflating the cuff.
2. **Use universal precautions.**
3. Have the nurse suction the oropharyngeal area.
4. Deflate the cuff partially or fully by inserting a 5- or 10-ml syringe into the cuff pilot balloon.
5. Have the patient swallow a barium bolus.
6. If aspiration occurs, have the patient cough to test the competency of clearing the airway.
7. Have the nurse suction the patient's tracheostomy tube if aspiration is not cleared with coughing.
8. Try other consistencies of barium.
9. Have the patient try therapeutic postures and swallowing compensation techniques.

10. Have the nurse suction as needed.
11. Reinflate the cuff after the test is finished.

CONSIDERATIONS BEFORE REQUESTING DIET ORDERS OR PERFORMING DYSPHAGIA THERAPY

Due to the fragile nature of tracheostomized and ventilator-dependent patients, special care should be exercised before beginning any oral feedings or treatment programs. Once a thorough evaluation has been performed, periodic reassessment will be necessary to modify the treatment program. It is important to always keep the following factors in mind when treating this population:

- If a patient silently aspirates one consistency and not others but appears at risk due to a delayed swallow response or pharyngeal pooling, consider recommending to restrict the patient to nothing by mouth (NPO). These patients may have a high incidence of inconsistent triggering of a swallow.
- There is heightened potential for impairments in pharyngeal propulsion and in airway protection.
- If the swallowing deficit is a result of prolonged intubation rather than neurologic damage and the patient is aspirating liquids, do not perform any type of therapy intervention that may cause the patient to produce more secretions (e.g., thermal stimulation).
- Do not practice hard swallows with the cuff inflated due to the possibility of tracheal irritation.

DIRECT AND INDIRECT TREATMENT METHODS

See Chapters 3 and 6 and Table 6.5 for a discussion on direct and indirect treatment methods for swallowing disorders.

REFERENCES

1. DeVita MA, Spierer L, Rundback MS. Swallowing disorders in patients with prolonged orotracheal intubation or tracheostomy tubes. Crit Care Med 1990;18:1328.
2. Logemann J. Evaluation and Treatment of Swallowing Disorders. San Diego: College-Hill, 1983;100.
3. Buchholz D. Neurologic evaluation of dysphagia. Dysphagia 1987;1:187.
4. Splaingard ML. Aspiration in rehabilitation patients: videofluoroscopy vs. bedside clinical assessment. Arch Phys Med Rehabil 1988;69:637.
5. Veis S, Logemann J. Swallowing disorders in persons with cerebrovascular accident. Arch Phys Med Rehabil 1985;66:372.
6. Sands JA. Incidence of pulmonary aspiration in intubated patients receiving enteral nutrition through wide- and narrow-bore nasogastric feeding tubes. Heart Lung 1991;20:75.
7. Dikeman FJ, Kazandjian MS. Communication and Swallowing Management of Tracheostomized and Ventilator-Dependent Adults. San Diego: Singular, 1995;251.
8. Petring OU, Adelhoj B, Jensen BN, et al. Prevention of silent aspiration due to leaks around cuffs of endotracheal tubes. Anesthesia 1986;65:777.

11

Managing Pediatric Feeding Problems

Low birth weight (LBW) and prematurity can negatively affect the swallowing and feeding performance of a newborn. LBW is defined as weighing less than 1,500 g at birth. Very low birth weight is defined as weighing less than 1,000 g at birth. A micropremie weighs less than 800 g at birth. Few infants weighing less than 500 g at birth survive. See Table 11.1 for a pounds-to-grams conversion chart.

The normal gestation period for humans is 38 weeks from fertilization, or 40 weeks from the mother's last menstrual cycle. An infant is unlikely to survive if born at a gestational period of less than 24 weeks, since significant respiratory and central nervous system development occurs from 24 to 32 weeks' gestation.

A child's corrected age should be considered when assessing any developmental behaviors up to 1 year of age. Some experts believe the corrected age should be considered up to 2 years of age. To calculate a premature infant's "corrected age," subtract the number of weeks the infant was premature (based on 40 weeks' gestation)

TABLE 11.1. Pounds-to-grams conversion chart*

Based on 1 oz = 28.3495 g

Pounds	Ounces							
	0	1	2	3	4	5	6	7
0	—	28	57	85	113	142	170	198
1	454	482	510	539	567	595	624	652
2	907	936	964	992	1,021	1,049	1,077	1,106
3	1,361	1,389	1,417	1,446	1,474	1,503	1,531	1,559
4	1,814	1,843	1,871	1,899	1,928	1,956	1,984	2,013
5	2,268	2,296	2,325	2,353	2,381	2,410	2,438	2,466
6	2,722	2,750	2,778	2,807	2,835	2,863	2,892	2,920
7	3,175	3,203	3,232	3,260	3,289	3,317	3,345	3,374
8	3,629	3,657	3,685	3,714	3,742	3,770	3,799	3,827
9	4,082	4,111	4,139	4,167	4,196	4,224	4,252	4,281
10	4,536	4,564	4,593	4,621	4,649	4,678	4,706	4,734
11	4,990	5,018	5,046	5,075	5,103	5,131	5,160	5,188
12	5,443	5,471	5,500	5,528	5,557	5,585	5,613	5,642
13	5,897	5,925	5,953	5,982	6,010	6,038	6,067	6,095
14	6,350	6,379	6,407	6,435	6,464	6,492	6,520	6,549

*For example, a 5- lb 7- oz baby weighs 2,466 g.

from his or her date of birth (i.e., chronologic age – prematurity in weeks = corrected age).

In addition to prematurity and LBW, other factors, such as central nervous system disorders, can lead to swallowing and feeding problems and poor growth in infants.

Central nervous system abnormalities, such as cerebral palsy or spina bifida, affect 3 of 1,000 births [1]. First and second branchial arch abnormalities also contribute to swallowing problems and are manifested in cleft palate, cleft lip, Treacher Collins syndrome, and Pierre Robin syndrome. Children born with Down's syndrome may have trouble with tongue coordination. Respiratory tract abnormalities (e.g.,

8	9	10	11	12	13	14	15	16
227	255	283	312	340	369	397	425	454
680	709	737	765	794	822	850	879	907
1,134	1,162	1,191	1,219	1,247	1,276	1,304	1,332	1,361
1,588	1,616	1,644	1,673	1,701	1,729	1,758	1,786	1,814
2,041	2,070	2,098	2,126	2,155	2,183	2,211	2,240	2,268
2,495	2,523	2,551	2,580	2,608	2,637	2,665	2,693	2,722
2,948	2,977	3,005	3,033	3,062	3,090	3,118	3,147	3,175
3,402	3,430	3,459	3,487	3,515	3,544	3,572	3,600	3,629
3,856	3,884	3,912	3,941	3,969	3,997	4,026	4,054	4,082
4,309	4,337	4,366	4,394	4,423	4,451	4,479	4,508	4,536
4,763	4,791	4,819	4,848	4,876	4,904	4,933	4,961	4,990
5,216	5,245	5,273	5,301	5,330	5,358	5,386	5,415	5,443
5,670	5,698	5,727	5,755	5,783	5,812	5,840	5,868	5,897
6,123	6,152	6,180	6,209	6,237	6,265	6,294	6,322	6,350
6,577	6,605	6,634	6,662	6,690	6,719	6,747	6,776	6,804

tracheoesophageal fistulas), esophageal abnormalities (e.g., esophageal atresia), stomach abnormalities, and cardiac defects are also seen in infants with oral-motor feeding problems. A glossary of neonatal intensive care unit terminology is provided at the end of the book to help the clinician in understanding the terminology found on a newborn's patient chart.

ASSESSMENT OF NEWBORNS

Apgar Scores

Apgar scores are the numerical rating of the vital signs of infants observed at 1 minute and 5 minutes after delivery [2]. Each attribute is scored 0, 1, or 2, and these scores are added together so that the maximum score is 10. Scores of 7–10 are considered good. Newborns with Apgar scores of 4–6 usually require resuscitation. Scores of 0–3 indicate acute distress. The Apgar newborn scoring system is provided in Table 11.2.

Brazelton Neonatal Behavioral Assessment Scale

A number of newborn behavioral examinations have been devised. The most widely used is the Brazelton Neonatal Behavioral Assessment Scale (NBAS). The NBAS allows quantitative estimation of the infant's neurologic intactness, adaptation to extrauterine life, primitive reflexes, state organization, self-regulatory ability, and interactive capacities from birth to 1 month. The scores do not correlate well with later development.

The examination takes approximately 30–45 minutes and requires extensive training before the examiner becomes proficient. The revised NBAS, which assesses 28 behavioral responses, tests and rates the infant on a 9-point scale. To assess the patterns of change, each infant should be examined at least two, but optimally three or more times. The first examination should be done after the stress of labor and delivery has begun to wear off, usually on the second or third day after birth. The second examination is best performed at 7–14 days, and the third at 1 month.

TABLE 11.2. The Apgar newborn scoring system

Sign	Points		
	0	1	2
Appearance (color)*	Pale or blue	Pink body, blue extremities	Pink overall
Pulse (heart rate in beats per minute)	Not detectable	Less than 100	More than 100
Grimace (reflex irritability)	No response to stimulation	Grimace, some motion	Lusty cry
Activity (muscle tone)	Flaccid (no or weak activity)	Some movement of extremities	Active motion, good flexion
Respiration (breathing)	None	Slow, irregular	Good (crying)

*In nonwhite infants, the color of the mucous membranes of the mouth, the whites of the eyes, and the lips, palms, hands, and soles of the feet will be examined.
Source: Reprinted with permission from V Apgar. The newborn (APGAR) scoring system: reflections and advice. Pediatr Clin North Am 1966;13:645.

Pediatric Swallowing Assessment

Assessment of a pediatric patient's swallowing should include the following:

I. Collect a detailed clinical history, including the following:

   A. Family and social history
   B. Prenatal history
   C. Birth history
   D. Pertinent medical history
   E. Appetite and diet

    F. Developmental status

    G. Parent-child interaction

    H. General health

    I. Abnormal swallowing patterns

  II. Assess the child's cognitive and motor milestones relevant to normal feeding (see Chapter 12).

 III. Assess the child's neurologic development. Observe child's posture, movements, general gross motor skills, and fine motor skills.

 IV. Assess the child's cranial nerve function (see Chapter 4).

  V. Examine the child's respiratory and heart rates at rest and during oral feedings. Note any audible pharyngeal secretions, stridor, and chest retractions.

 VI. Assess the child's reflexes (Table 11.3).

 VII. Assess the child's oral-motor function.

VIII. Observe feeding. Note nature, severity, positional problems, and possible complications of the dysphagia. See Table 11.4 for signs of stress in premature infants during oral feedings.

FEEDING NEWBORNS IN THE NEONATAL INTENSIVE CARE UNIT

Management of Swallowing Problems of Nonorally Fed Infants

Oral-motor stimulation and treatment are of particular importance to children who are being fed nonorally in that they facilitate the transition to oral feedings and pre-

TABLE 11.3. Infant oral reflexes

Reflex	Stimulus	Age of appearance	Age of disappearance	Pass	Fail
Rooting	Stroke front of lips	Birth	3–6 mos	Mouth opens or suckling begins	Mouth does not open, no suckling
Suckling	Nipple in mouth	Birth	6–12 mos	Suckling begins; suck is strong and immediate	No suckling begins; suck is weak
Swallowing	Bolus of food in pharynx	Birth	Persists from birth	Swallow is immediate after three to four sucks	Swallow not seen after seven or more sucks
Tongue	Touch tongue or lips	Birth	12–18 mos	Suckle-swallow reaction	No suckling response
Bite	Pressure on gums	Birth	9–12 mos	No bite felt	Bite felt
Gag	Touch tongue or pharynx	Birth	Persists from birth	Gag not observed or weak gag may be seen	Gag observed

Source: Adapted from RJ Love, WG Webb. Neurology for the Speech-Language Pathologist. Boston: Butterworth–Heinemann, 1992;265; and B Landry. Neonatal Assessment for Feeding and State Organization. Boulder, CO: NAFSO, 1990.

TABLE 11.4. Signs of stress in premature infants

Autonomic behaviors
    Color changes (any color changes, pallor, cyanosis, or duskiness)
    Note baseline color.
    Decrease or increase in heart rate (bradycardia or tachycardia) (Average heartbeats per minute in a neonate is 120–160.)
    Increase or decrease in respirations (tachypnea, apnea)
    Decrease in oxygen saturation
    Gagging or coughing
    Spitting up
Motor behaviors
    Straightening or tensing the limbs
    Stiffening body or arching back
    Flailed fingers
    Jerky movements
    Flaccidity of trunk, neck, face, or extremities
    Variable tone
    Tongue extensions
State behaviors
    Irritability
    Frantic activity
    Frowns or grimaces
    Sudden fatigue or weak state
    Sudden onset of disorganized sleepiness or drowsiness
    Looks of worry, panic, or hyperalertness
    Fussiness or crying
    Change in state of alertness
    Yawning
    Averting eye contact
    Covering face with hand
    Flaccid face, tongue extensions

Source: Adapted from H Als et al. Manual for the Assessment of Preterm Infant's Behavior (APIB). In HE Fitzgerald, BM Lester, MW Yogman (eds), Theory and Research in Behavioral Pediatrics (Vol 1). New York: Plenum, 1982;65.

vent oral aversion behaviors. An oral-motor treatment approach is used to encourage coordinated timing and sufficient muscle strength for food and liquid to be swallowed safely without aspiration (Table 11.5).

Management of Suck and Swallow Problems of Orally Fed Infants

When an infant is medically stable, the progression to feeding is an individualized program. Some of the signs that an infant is ready to begin oral feedings include the ability to move the hands to the mouth or face and the ability to coordinate breathing with sucking and swallowing. Management suggestions for pediatric feeding problems are listed in Table 11.6.

When feeding a newborn, the clinician should ensure optimal feeding conditions. An infant who is agitated, overstimulated, or crying will not feed well. Methods to calm the infant are listed below.

- Limit or tone down stimuli.
- Keep room light dim.
- Present one stimulus at a time.
- Contain or swaddle the infant.
- Rock the infant with even rhythmical movements.
- Gently bounce and rock the infant up and down while standing.
- Hold the infant gently but firmly.

TABLE 11.5. Techniques to improve oral motor function in infants

Goal	Technique
To reduce bite reflex	Rub the infant's gums in four quadrants, and wait for swallow.
To reduce gag	Use firm pressure when touching the infant.
	Massage the infant's cheeks in small circles.
	Gradually and firmly stroke the infant's tongue from back to front at midline.
	Use finger and place some milk in the buccal pocket then massage cheek.
	Gradually press a tongue blade from the anterior to the posterior tongue.
To improve root and open reflex	Touch the infant's lips with nipple of a bottle or finger and pause to allow mouth to open.
	Place small amount of fluid on lip and wait for the infant's mouth to open and possibly suck.
	Press your thumb firmly in the palm of the baby's hand.
To increase hand-to-mouth coordination	Swaddle the infant.
	Keep the infant's shoulders and arms rolled forward.
	Assist the infant's hand to the mouth.
To reduce oral hypersensitivity	Maintain deep sustained pressure in and around the mouth by the caregiver's or infant's hand.
To improve consistent sucking rhythm	With fingertip at the infant's midtongue, stroke toward front with pressure down on tongue 4–6 times at 1–2 strokes per second; hold the infant's tongue. Repeat after several seconds.
To reduce sucking incoordination, to encourage more sucking, or to improve cheek tone	Place a pacifier or finger in the infant's mouth. Hold it in place if infant tends to push it out.
To improve suck-swallow-respiratory sequencing in infants not safe for oral feeding	Dampen a swab with water, formula, or breast milk. Place the swab at the infant's midtongue, and stroke with downward pressure to release minimal amount of liquid. Repeat as tolerated in a pleasurable way.

To improve jaw control and movement	Stroke or massage forward from back of the infant's jaw to front.
	Apply quick, firm taps under the infant's chin.
	Flex the infant's body position.
	When the infant is ready for oral feeding, stabilize his or her jaw by placing your finger under the infant's jaw.
To improve normal tongue position and movement	Stroke the infant's tongue from back to front at midline and sides.
	Have the infant suck on your finger when non-nutritive sucking; if the tongue is humped, apply firm pressure to the midtongue blade.
	To continue tongue movement, apply firm strokes under the infant's chin and move finger from back to front.
To improve lip movement	Massage the infant's cheeks and lips.
	Gently tap or stroke around the infant's lips.
	Provide jaw support.
	Keep infant's head flexed forward and chin tucked.

Source: Adapted from B Landry. Neonatal Assessment for Feeding and State Organization. Boulder, CO: NAFSO, 1990; and JC Arvedson, L Brodsky. Pediatric Swallowing and Feeding: Assessment and Management. San Diego: Singular, 1993;345.

An infant who is lethargic and cannot remain awake long enough to complete a feeding is at nutritional risk as well. Methods to facilitate arousal in an infant are listed below.

- Apply deep pressure to the soles of the feet, palms of the hands, or the back.
- Rock the infant in uneven rhythms in any direction.
- Rock the infant from side-to-side or in a rotary direction while supporting the head.

TABLE 11.6. Suggestions for the management of pediatric feeding problems

Pediatric feeding problem	Symptoms	Management suggestions
Weak suck or decreased lip seal	Nipple can be removed too easily from infant's mouth Oral loss of liquids around the nipple Minimal amount of bubbles generated around the nipple Insufficient energy to consume sufficient quantity of food in a reasonable length of time	Apply pressure to the orbicularis oris to assist lip closure. Tug at nipple as though pulling it out of the infant's mouth (may smooth out and strengthen the suck). Thicken liquid (rice cereal). Adjust nipple opening.
Oral-pharyngeal dysphagia or pharyngeal dysmotility	Excessive coughing, choking, tachypnea, or gagging Delayed swallow Poor weight gain Wet or gargled vocal sounds Multiple swallows per bolus	Pursue further objective testing (i.e., videofluoroscopy) to determine etiology of swallowing dysfunction.
Suck and swallow incoordination	Coughing, choking, or gagging Decrease in respirations Aversion to feedings	Stroke hyoid musculature toward sternum. Gradually introduce liquid (using a finger, pacifier, cotton swab, or cheesecloth that is dipped in liquid and placed in mouth). Change nipple to obtain optimal flow. Bypass nippling to spoon and cup.

Pediatric feeding problem	Symptoms	Management suggestions
		Allow breaks to allow infant to reorganize breathing.
Oral hypersensitivity due to tube feedings or oral suctioning	Aversion to nippling or other oral stimulation Irritability with oral stimulation	Apply deep sustained pressure in and around mouth with your hand or the infant's hand.
Oral hyposensitivity	Lackadaisical feeding	Use firm but gentle stroking around the infant's mouth and on tongue.
Poor appetite	Insufficient oral intake at feedings	Feed when the infant is hungry (demand schedule). Reduce tube feedings during daytime and supplement at night.
Gastroesophageal reflux	Vomiting Esophagitis Mucosal inflammation or ulceration Coughing Apnea	Feed the infant thickened liquids. Elevate the infant's head in the prone position (not clearly supported). Medical or surgical treatment is probably necessary.

Source: Adapted from JC Arvedson, L Brodsky. Pediatric Swallowing and Feeding: Assessment and Management. San Diego: Singular, 1993;348.

Most of an infant's actions during feeding are related to airway maintenance or airway protection. If an infant is unable to maintain his or her airway, he or she will show signs of distress. Not responding to these signs can lead to an infant's not feeding well or can lead to respiratory distress.

Signs of poor regulation of breathing during feeding may be reflected by the following:

- Decreased endurance and respiratory fatigue
- Tachypnea
- Nasal flaring, blanching of the nares (nares turn white), or both
- Chin tugging
- "Catch breaths" (quick shallow breaths)
- High-pitched crowing sounds

Signs of difficulty in regulating swallowing during feeding may be reflected by the following:

- Drooling
- Gulping
- Gurgling sounds in the pharynx
- Double swallowing
- Coughing, choking, or both

MANAGEMENT OF CLEFT LIP AND PALATE INFANTS

Cleft lip and cleft palate are two of the most frequently occurring congenital anomalies. The incidence of clefting of some kind in the white population is approximately 1 in 600 births. The incidence is higher in Asian populations and lower in black populations [3]. If cleft lip or cleft palate is detected at birth, there will be management issues concerning appearance, dental and jaw relationships, swallowing and nutrition, and speech and hearing. The most immediate concerns are swallowing and nutrition.

Definitions and Types of Cleft Lips and Palates

A *cleft lip* is a congenital deformity of the upper lip that varies from a notching to a complete division of the lip. The alveolar process and palate may or may not be involved. A combination of cleft lip and cleft palate occurs more frequently than either condition occurs separately. There are several types of cleft lips:

- In a *unilateral cleft lip*, the cleft is either on the right or left side of the upper lip and extends from the vermilion border toward the nostril.
- In a *median cleft lip*, a vertical cleft extends through the center of the upper lip.
- In a *bilateral cleft lip*, the cleft extends from the vermilion border of the upper lip toward both the right and left nostrils.

A *cleft palate* is a congenital fissure in the median line of the palate that can extend through the uvula, soft palate, and hard palate. A cleft lip may or may not be involved. There are several types of cleft palates:

- In a *bilateral cleft palate*, the palate on the right and left sides fails to fuse with the nasal partition or septum.

- In a *complete or total cleft palate*, the cleft extends from the lip through the alveolar process, hard palate, and soft palate.
- In an *incomplete, partial, or subtotal cleft palate*, the cleft can be limited to the lip, alveolar process, hard palate, soft palate, or a combination of these structures.
- In a *submucous cleft palate*, the surface tissues of the hard or soft palate unite but the underlying bone or muscle tissues do not. It may occur alone or in structures adjacent to incomplete clefts. It is characterized by a bifid uvula, zona pellucida (in which the muscles are absent under the soft palatal mucosa), or a notched or V-shaped hard palate. An occult submucous cleft palate can occur, however, in the absence of all of these.
- An *occult submucous cleft palate* is characterized by velopharyngeal insufficiency secondary to absent musculus uvulae [1].
- In a *unilateral cleft palate*, the palate fuses to the vertical nasal septum on one side only.

Diagrams of the types of cleft lips and palates are provided in Figure 11.1.

Speech and language in a cleft palate child may or may not be symptomatic. Some characteristics found in cleft palate include the following:

- Hypernasality
- Inaccurate articulation and frequent substitutions of nasal, pharyngeal, and glottal sounds

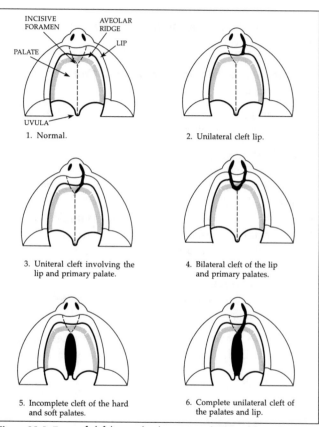

INCISIVE FORAMEN
AVEOLAR RIDGE
LIP
PALATE
UVULA

1. Normal.

2. Unilateral cleft lip.

3. Uniteral cleft involving the lip and primary palate.

4. Bilateral cleft of the lip and primary palates.

5. Incomplete cleft of the hard and soft palates.

6. Complete unilateral cleft of the palates and lip.

Figure 11.1. Types of cleft lips and palates. Ventral views of the palate, alveolar ridge, lip, and nose illustrate the various degrees of cleft palate and cleft lip. (Modified from J Langman. Medical Embryology [3rd ed]. Baltimore: Williams & Wilkins, 1975.)

- Nasal emission during production of fricative sounds
- Delayed development of language skills

Management of Feeding Problems in Cleft Palate and Cleft Lip Infants

Feeding problems found in infants with cleft palate or cleft lip include the following:

- Reduced sucking efficiency due to an inability to develop negative intraoral pressure
- Incoordination of sucking and swallowing, causing choking
- Choking due to an inconsistent or rapid liquid flow rate
- Nasal reflux or nasal regurgitation due to an inability to seal off the nasal cavity
- Excessive amounts of ingested air, which necessitates frequent burping
- Airway obstruction due to a small mandible, glossoptosis, or both

Guidelines for oral feeding of infants with cleft palate are found in Table 11.7.

TABLE 11.7. Basic oral feeding guidelines for infants with cleft palate

Attributes	Guidelines
Position	Place the infant in an upright position (60–90 degrees), and provide good trunk, neck, and head support (this prevents milk from coming out of the baby's nose).
	Help the baby form a seal around the nipple by holding the baby's cheeks close to the nipple with your index finger and thumb. Use your middle finger to support the baby's lower jaw.
Nipple	Use a cross-cut nipple that compresses easily.
	Use a soft nipple with a thin wall that compresses easily.
	The use of a wide, flat (Nuk or orthodontic) nipple is optional.
	The nipple should help strengthen and develop orofacial muscles without excessive effort.
Container	Use a flexible plastic squeeze bottle.
	Use a rigid container that is cut out to allow for squeezing of bag or liner.
	Use the Haberman feeder.
Liquid flow	Make sure that the flow is easy and steady.
	Make sure that the flow is slow enough to prevent choking.
	Ensure the flow is not too fast so that normal swallowing can occur.
Timing	Burp frequently during feeding.
	Allow 20–30 min for total feeding.
	Feed at 2- to 4-hr intervals.
	Keep infant upright for 20 to 30 min after each feeding.
Hygiene	Keep infant's mouth, lip, and nose area clean.

Source: Adapted from JC Arvedson, L Brodsky. Pediatric Swallowing and Feeding: Assessment and Management. San Diego: Singular, 1993;425.

REFERENCES

1. Arvedson JC, Brodsky L. Pediatric Swallowing and Feeding: Assessment and Management. San Diego: Singular, 1993;24,249,417.

2. Apgar V. The newborn (APGAR) scoring system: reflections and advice. Pediatr Clin North Am, 1966;13:645.
3. Moller KT, Starr CD (eds). Cleft Palate: Interdisciplinary Issues and Treatment. Austin, TX: PRO-ED. 1993;229.

SUGGESTED READING

Als H, et al. Manual for the Assessment of Preterm Infant's Behavior (APIB). In HE Fitzgerald, BM Lester, MW Yogman (eds), Theory and Research in Behavioral Pediatrics (Vol 1). New York: Plenum, 1982;65.

Billeaud FP. Communication Disorders in Infants and Toddlers. Boston: Andover, 1993.

Brazelton TB. Behavioral Competence. In GB Avery, MA Fletcher, MG MacDonald (eds), Neonatology: Pathophysiology and Management of the Newborn (4th ed). Philadelphia: Lippincott, 1994;289.

Landry B. Neonatal Assessment for Feeding and State Organization. Boulder, CO: NAFSO, 1990.

Love RJ, Webb WG. Neurology for the Speech-Language Pathologist (3rd ed). Boston: Butterworth-Heinemann, 1996.

Nicolosi L, Harryman E, Kresheck J. Terminology of Communication Disorders: Speech-Language-Hearing (3rd ed). Baltimore: Williams & Wilkins, 1989.

12

Child Development

DEVELOPMENTAL SEQUENCES OF MOTOR AND LANGUAGE BEHAVIOR

Each child is an individual, and what is considered "normal" covers a wide range. Premature infants tend to reach milestones later than full-term infants of the same birth age. Premature children will often achieve milestones closer to their corrected age or even later. *Corrected age* is the age that the infant would be if he or she had been born at term.

The milestones listed in Table 12.1 are based on what approximately 90% of children have mastered at a particular age [1, 2]. A child may not necessarily reach each milestone at the listed age but may still be developing at a completely normal rate for that child.

TABLE 12.1. Milestones in childhood development

Age	Motor/sensory development	Receptive/expressive language development	Pragmatics
Birth to 3 mos	Lifts head briefly when on stomach or a flat surface Moves arms and legs on both sides of the body equally well Focuses on objects within 8–15 ins. Begins hand-to-mouth movements Plays with a rattle	Maintains brief eye contact during feeding Smiles in response to your smile Quiets to a familiar voice Responds to sound—reflex smiling or vocalizing to mother's voice Cries to get attention Vocalizes in other ways than crying (e.g., cooing and vowel vocalizations) Gives vocal expression to feelings of pleasure Laughs out loud	Cries to get attention Shows interest in people, not objects Seeks to make eye contact
3–6 mos	Lifts head 90 degrees when on stomach Reaches for objects Bangs objects in play Uses both hands to hold a bottle Rolls over Holds head steady when	Uses sound to get attention Smiles spontaneously Smiles at faces Turns head toward a voice Babbles Takes turns vocalizing	Maintains eye contact Vocalizes in response to vocalization Imitates facial expressions Produces different cries for different reasons

Age			
6–9 mos	upright Raises chest, supported by arms, when on stomach Keeps head level with body when pulled to a sitting position Feeds self a cracker Bears some weight on legs when held upright Sits without support Passes a block from one hand to the other Rakes up small objects and picks them up in fist Looks for a dropped object Works to get an out-of-reach toy	Stops crying when spoken to Whines purposefully Attempts to interact with an adult Vocalizes four different syllables Vocalizes a two-syllable combination Attends to music or singing Waves bye-bye Responds to "no" Stops activity when name is called Attends to pictures Vocalizes to get attention	Exchanges gestures Uses gestures and vocalizations to protest Vocalizes or shouts to get attention
9–12 mos	Drinks from a cup held by a caregiver (9–10 mos) Stands holding on to someone or something Pulls up to standing position from sitting	Objects if you try to take a toy away Says "mama" or "dada" meaningfully	Vocalizes to call others Vocalizes when another person calls Indicates a desire for a

TABLE 12.1. (continued)

Age	Motor/sensory development	Receptive/expressive language development	Pragmatics
	Uses pincer grasp for finger feeding (10–11 mos) Gets into a sitting position from stomach Picks up a small object with any part of thumb or finger Walks holding on to furniture Holds cup with two hands	Plays peekaboo Points to or looks at objects to indicate awareness Imitates consonant and vowel combinations Imitates nonspeech sounds Uses one to two words spontaneously Follows simple commands occasionally Understands simple questions Identifies two body parts on self	change in activities
12–15 mos	Pulls up to standing position Gets into a sitting position Walks holding on to furniture Claps hands Stands alone Puts an object into a container	Follows one-step commands during play Will say words upon request Points to two action words in pictures Identifies three body parts on self or a doll Shakes head "no"	Imitates other children Responds to children's vocalizations Initiates turn-taking Uses more words during turn-taking

Age			
	Walks well Bends over and picks up an object Feeds others	Has an 8- to 10-word vocabulary Imitates three animal sounds Asks to have needs met Uses true words within jargon-like utterances	Points to, shows, or gives objects Controls the behavior of self and others Uses words to protest
15–18 mos	Imitates activities Scribbles Drinks from a cup	Finds familiar objects not in sight Understands 50 words Has a 15-word vocabulary Can name five to seven familiar objects upon request Identifies objects by category Can identify six body parts on doll	
18–21 mos	Dumps an object in imitation Uses a spoon Runs Builds a tower of two blocks Imitates housework activities Takes off an article of clothing	Uses single words frequently Imitates two- and three-word phrases Uses two-word phrases occasionally Understands the meaning of action words Identifies pictures when named	Engages in adult-like dialogue Uses words and vocalizations during pretend play Uses words to interact with others Takes turns talking during conversation

TABLE 12.1. (continued)

Age	Motor/sensory development	Receptive/expressive language development	Pragmatics
21–24 mos	Walks up steps Kicks a small ball forward Feeds a doll Builds a tower of four cubes Puts away toys on request Assembles toys and objects	Follows a two-step related command Chooses one object from a group of five on request Uses two-word phrases frequently and three-word phrases occasionally Uses 50 words Refers to self by name MLU = 1.25–1.50	Engages in parallel play Imitates simple actions
24–27 mos	Pretends to write Pretends to talk on the telephone Wipes hands and face Uses most toys appropriately	Recognizes family members' names Understands the concept of 1 Understands size concepts Uses three-word phrases frequently Imitates words upon request Asks for assistance Uses action words	Copies domestic activities in play Initiates own play activities Engages in simple make-believe activities Has tantrums when frustrated

		No items at this age level
27–30 mos	Puts on an article of clothing Jumps	MLU = 1.5–2.0 Responds to simple questions Identifies four objects by function Uses two sentence types Able to name at least one color Refers to self by pronoun
30–33 mos	Brushes teeth with help Builds a six-block tower Performs longer sequences of play activities Acts out familiar routines	MLU = 2.0–2.5 Follows two-step unrelated commands Answers yes or no questions correctly Uses plurals Uses prepositions Understands concepts of one and all Able to state first and last name	Looks for missing toys Dresses with supervision and some help
33–36 mos	Washes and dries hands Throws a ball overhand Draws with a crayon Can unzip clothing Can walk a straight line and maintain balance	Speaks and is understood half the time Carries on a conversation of two or three sentences	Begins cooperative play

TABLE 12.1. (continued)

Age	Motor/sensory development	Receptive/expressive language development	Pragmatics
48 mos	Hops on one foot for two to three hops Shows hand preference for drawing	Comprehends 1,500 words Uses four- to five-word sentences Uses compound and complex sentences	Separates from mother easily
60 mos	Colors somewhat within lines	Comprehends most concepts of space, time, quantity, and sequence Has a vocabulary of 2,500 words Uses five- to seven-word sentences Uses all types of sentences Can define some simple words Follows three-step commands	Enjoys group play
72 mos	Most gross motor skills are similar to an adult's	Can tell a familiar story when prompted to do so	No items at this age level

MLU = mean length of utterance.
Source: Modified from VK Frankenburg, JB Dodds. Denver Developmental Screening II. Denver: Ladoca Project and Publishing Foundation, 1990; and L Rossetti. The Rossetti Infant-Toddler Language Scale. East Moline, IL: LinguiSystems, 1990.

GENERAL GUIDELINES OF SPEECH SOUND DEVELOPMENT

Table 12.2 shows the ages at which sounds begin to emerge and the ages at which 75% of all English-speaking children master the sounds. Table 12.3 shows the ages at which 75% of American English-speaking children master consonant clusters [3, 4]. It is important to remember that there may be slight variations within cultures. It is up to the individual clinician to familiarize himself or herself with the cultural norms for the groups served.

TABLE 12.2. General guidelines of speech sound development

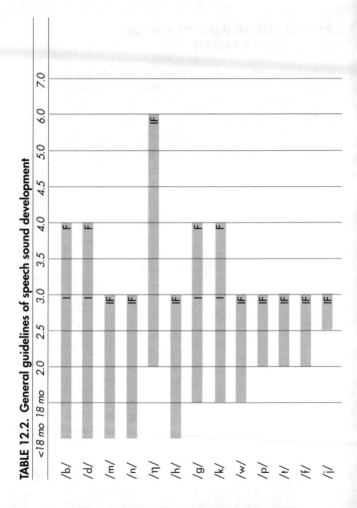

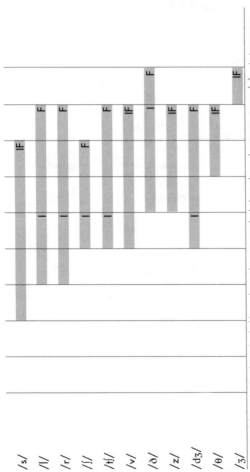

/s/ /l/ /r/ /ʃ/ /tʃ/ /v/ /ð/ /z/ /dʒ/ /θ/ /ʒ/

Note: The left-hand side of the shaded bars shows the age at which the indicated consonant sounds begin to emerge in American English. The righthand side shows the earliest age at which 75% of American English-speaking children produce each test sound element correctly. The I (initial) and the F (final) indicate the earliest age at which the sound is usually mastered in the initial and final positions.

Source: Adapted from A Smit, L Hand, J Freilinger, et al. The Iowa Articulation Norms Project and its Nebraska replication. J Speech Hear Disord 1990;55:779; and EK Sander. When are speech sounds learned? J Speech Hear Disord 1972;37:55.

Table 12.3. The age at which 75% of American children acquire American English consonant clusters in initial word positions

Age of acquisition (yrs)	Consonant cluster
3.5	/tw/, /kw/
4.5	/gl/
5.0	/sp/, /st/, /sk/, /sm/, /bl/
5.5	/sn/, /sw/, /pl/, /kl/, /fl/, /tr/, /kr/
6.0	/pr/, /br/, /dr/, /gr/, /fr/
7.0	/sl/, /θr/, /skw/, /spl/
8.0	/spr/, /str/, /skr/

Source: Modified from A Smit, L Hand, J Frelinger, et al. The Iowa Articulation Norms Project and Its Nebraska Replication. J Speech Hear Disord 1990;55:779.

REFERENCES

1. Rossetti L. The Rossetti Infant-Toddler Language Scale. East Moline, IL: LinguiSystems, 1990;1.
2. Frankenburg WK, Dodds JB. Denver Developmental Screening II. Denver: Ladoca Project and Publishing Foundation, 1990.
3. Smit A, Hand L, Frelinger J, et al. The Iowa Articulation Norms Project and its Nebraska replication. J Speech Hear Disord 1990;55:779.
4. Sander EK. When are speech sounds learned? J Speech Hear Disord 1972;37:55.

13

Dentition

The teeth play important roles in articulation by serving as markers for the tongue positioning and by modifying the air stream for various speech sounds. Both misalignment of the upper and lower teeth and incorrect positioning of individual teeth can contribute to poor articulation of certain sounds. Humans have 20 deciduous teeth ("baby" teeth) and 32 permanent teeth. The standard numbering system for the teeth is provided in Figure 13.1. This system should be used in identifying and reporting tooth alignment and positioning issues that may be contributing to poor articulation.

A misalignment of the upper (maxillary) and lower (mandibular) teeth is called a *malocclusion* and is normally determined by the position of the upper first molars (permanent) relative to the positions of the lower first molars (permanent). In normal occlusion ("bite"), the mesiobuccal cusp of the maxillary first molar should fit into the buccal groove of the mandibular first molar without any other tooth deviation [1]. The types of malocclusions are discussed in the following sections.

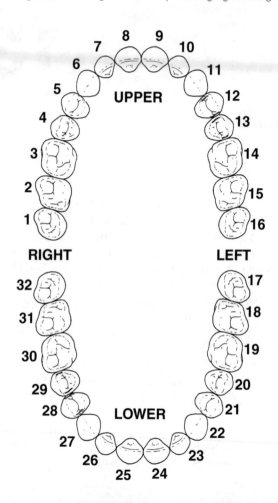

1. Upper right third molar
2. Upper right second molar
3. Upper right first molar
4. Upper right second bicuspid
5. Upper right first bicuspid
6. Upper right canine
7. Upper right lateral incisor
8. Upper right central incisor
9. Upper left central incisor
10. Upper left lateral incisor
11. Upper left canine
12. Upper left first bicuspid
13. Upper left second bicuspid
14. Upper left first molar
15. Upper left second molar
16. Upper left third molar
17. Lower left third molar
18. Lower left second molar
19. Lower left first molar
20. Lower left second bicuspid
21. Lower left first bicuspid
22. Lower left canine
23. Lower left lateral incisor
24. Lower left central incisor
25. Lower right central incisor
26. Lower right lateral incisor
27. Lower right canine
28. Lower right first bicuspid
29. Lower right second bicuspid
30. Lower right first molar
31. Lower right second molar
32. Lower right third molar

Figure 13.1. Standard numbering for the teeth. The numbering system begins with the back upper right tooth (the third molar) and progresses forward and around to the back upper left. The numbering then progresses from the back lower left around to the back lower right.

Neutroclusion (Angle's classification, class I)

In neutroclusion, there is a normal anteroposterior relationship between the maxillary and mandibular dental arches; however, there may be possible anterior deviations of individual tooth positions, missing teeth, and tooth size discrepancies.

Distoclusion (Angle's classification, class II)

In distoclusion, the lower dental arch is in a posterior relation to the upper dental arch. There are two types of distoclusion. The first, a *division I distoclusion*, occurs when the maxillary incisor teeth protrude in a facioversion or overjet malposition. This can result in an excessive overbite. The second, a *division II distoclusion*, occurs when the mandibular dental arch assumes an irregular curve, with supraversion of the mandibular incisor teeth, and the maxillary dental arch is wider than normal. This results in a closed bite.

Mesioclusion (Angle's classification, class III)

In mesioclusion, the first permanent mandibular molar teeth are anterior in their relationship with the maxillary first molar teeth, causing the mandibular incisor teeth to protrude and create an underbite. The maxillary dental arch is constricted and the tongue frequently rests on the floor of the mouth. A prognathic jaw can result from an extreme case of a mesioclusion.

TEETH MALPOSITIONS

The incorrect positioning of individual teeth is referred to as *malposition*. Malpositions can interfere with both articulation and mastication. Malpositions can also affect the patient's cosmetic appearance. Malpositions can contribute to malocclusions and can result from malocclusions as well. The types of teeth malpositions are listed below.

Axioversion — The slanting of teeth along an improper axis

Buccoversion — The slanting of teeth toward the lips or cheeks; also known as facioversion

Closed bite — Extension of upper teeth beyond the normal line of occlusion; also known as supraversion

Cross-bite — A condition in which the maxillary and mandibular teeth are not aligned vertically with each other; one or more teeth may be abnormally malpositioned buccally, lingually, or labially with the opposing tooth or teeth

Distoversion — The tipping or slanting of teeth away from the middle of the dental arch

Facioversion — The slanting of teeth toward the lips or cheeks; also known as buccoversion and labioversion

Infraversion — A condition in which teeth have not erupted sufficiently to reach the proper line of occlusion

Jumbling — The overcrowding of teeth resulting in their being overlapped or massed together

Labioversion — The slanting of teeth toward the lips or cheeks; also known as facioversion

Linguoversion — The slanting or tipping of teeth toward the tongue or the inside of the mouth

Mesioversion — The slanting or tipping of teeth toward the midline of the dental arch

Open bite — A condition in which the anterior upper teeth appear to be too short to reach the midline; the posterior teeth may have grown past the midline point; thumb sucking may also be a contributing factor

Overbite — Excessive supraversion or closed bite

Overjet — A condition in which the upper maxillary teeth extend past the normal line of occlusion and in the direction of the lips

Supernumerary teeth — Teeth in excess of the usual number in the dental arch

Supraversion — Extension of upper teeth beyond the normal line of occlusion; also known as closed bite

Torsiversion — The rotation of teeth along their vertical axis

Transversion — A condition in which teeth are in the wrong sequential order along the dental arch, even though they may be inclined properly

Underbite — A condition in which the mandibular teeth protrude and overlap the maxillary teeth that results in the
appearance of the mandible jutting forward

REFERENCES

1. Proffit WR. Contemporary Orthodontics. St. Louis: Mosby, 1986;3.

SUGGESTED READING

Nicolosi L, Harryman E, Kresheck J. Terminology of Communication
Disorders Speech-Language-Hearing (3rd ed). Baltimore: Williams
& Wilkins, 1989.

14

Fluency Disorders

WHAT IS DYSFLUENCY?

A *fluency disorder* is an involuntary repetition, prolongation, or blockage of a word or part of a word that a person is trying to say. The exact etiology of fluency disorders is still not known. Both organic and functional explanations have been examined but not proven. Fluency disorders, however, are thought to result from the interaction of multiple physiologic and psychological factors. Most often the problem is developmental in nature, beginning during the early years of a child's speech and language development; however, some cases of neurologic dysfluency have resulted from brain lesion.

Many children go through a normal period of dysfluency. It is therefore important to assess the distinction between normal and abnormal dysfluency (Table 14.1). Often, a fluency disorder begins gradually during the period when a child is acquiring language at a rapid rate, generally between 2 and 5 years of age. The critical period of what may become a lifetime pattern of dysfluency generally occurs between 5 and 7 years of age. Many factors influ-

TABLE 14.1. Guidelines for differentiating normal from abnormal dysfluency

Behavior	Abnormal dysfluency	Normal dysfluency
Syllable repetitions		
Number of unit repetitions per word [2]	At least three unit repetitions per part-word repetition, audible silent prolongations, and broken words predominate (e.g., "b-b-b-ball")	No more than two unit repetitions per part-word repetition (e.g., "b-b-ball")
Frequency of dysfluencies (per 100 words)	At least 10 dysfluencies per every 100 words spoken, or three within-word dysfluencies per 100 words spoken	Nine or fewer dysfluencies per every 100 words spoken
Rate of repetition	Faster than fluent speech	Same as fluent speech
Overall rate of speech	Irregular, inconsistently fast and slow	Consistent and smooth
Schwa vowel substituted for other vowels	Often present (e.g., "buh-buh-buh-beet")	Absent or rare (e.g., "bee-bee-beet")
Airflow	Often interrupted	Rarely interrupted
Vocal tension	Often apparent	Absent
Clustering [1]	Two types of fluency breaks within a word	One type of fluency break per word
Prolongations		
Duration	Longer than 1 sec	Less than 1 sec
Frequency	More than one per 100 words	Less than one per 100 words
Regularity	Uneven or interrupted	Smooth
Tension	Present in laryngeal or vocal areas	Absent

When voiced	May show rise in pitch during fluency breaks	No pitch rise
When unvoiced	Interrupted airflow	Airflow present
Termination of fluency breaks	Sudden	Gradual
Silent pauses		
Within the word boundary	May be present	Absent
Prior to speech attempt	Unusually long	Not marked
After the dysfluency	May be present	Absent
Phonation		
Inflections	Restricted; monotoned	Normal
Phonatory arrest	May be present	Absent
Vocal fry	May be present	Usually absent
Articulating postures	May be inappropriate	Appropriate
Primary type of dysfluencies	Part-word repetitions, audible-silent prolongations, and broken words predominate	Whole-word, phrase repetitions, interjections, and revisions predominate
Reactions to Stress	More broken words	Normal dysfluencies
Evidence of Awareness		
Phonemic consistency	May be present	Absent
Frustration	May be present	Absent
Postponements	May be present	Absent
Eye contact	May waver	Normal

Source: Modified from C Van Riper. The Nature of Stuttering (2nd ed). Englewood Cliffs, NJ: Prentice-Hall, 1982.

ence whether a child will have incipient dysfluencies or develop a fluency disorder. Some of these factors include any history of dysfluency in the family, family attitudes toward the dysfluent behavior, and the communicative environment and culture in which the child is raised [1].

Perhaps as many as 50–80% of children who begin to have dysfluencies recover without formal assistance. Of those children who continue to have abnormal dysfluencies, the sooner effective help is provided, the better the child's chances for achieving fluent speech. Treatment should include family counseling to provide parents with information about their child's dysfluency and strategies to help their child. Treatment for young children is often highly effective. If the abnormal dysfluencies continue after puberty, they usually persist throughout the individual's life.

As important as the dysfluencies themselves is the impact the dysfluency has on the patient's life. It is important to assess what the patient does and does not do because of the dysfluencies. The behaviors seen in the therapy room may not be representative of what is occurring outside of therapy. A patient in a relaxed, accepting environment may show great variability in the behavior causing the concern.

DYSFLUENCY EVALUATION

Evaluation Instructions for Patients Ages 3–10

1. Video- or audiotape a portion of the session or have the patient or parent bring a videotape that illustrates

the dysfluent behavior causing the concern. Time only the patient's speaking and reading time.

2. Count the dysfluencies by the syllable or word and not by dysfluent event.

3. Use a stopwatch and enter the patient's speaking time beside each task. Enter the total speaking time in minutes on the line at the end of the evaluation.

4. Count the total number of words spoken by the patient for each task and enter them on the appropriate line.

5. Count the number of dysfluent words spoken by the patient for each task and enter them on the appropriate line.

6. In order to obtain the number of dysfluent words per minute, for each task, section, or both, divide the total number of dysfluent words by the total time taken to speak.

7. For each task, section, or both, divide the total number of dysfluent words spoken by the total number of words spoken. Subtract the quotient from 100 to obtain percent of fluent speech. For example:

Dysfluent words = 5
Total words = 20
$5 \div 20 = 0.25$
$1.00 - 0.25 = 0.75$, or 75% fluency

Evaluation Instructions for Patients Ages 10 and Older

1. Obtain general background information, family history, educational history, personal interests, and occupational interests.

2. Obtain therapy background information, previous therapy, techniques used, success rate, and reason for therapy termination.

3. Discuss why the client is seeking therapy at this time. Has his or her dysfluent behavior recently changed?

4. Discuss patient's perception of the severity of his or her dysfluency.

5. Have the patient rate the variability in the dysfluent behavior.

6. Assess whether the patient can describe his or her dysfluent behavior and other people's reactions to it.

7. Have the patient explain what behaviors he or she exhibits because of the dysfluencies (secondary behaviors).

8. Have the patient describe how the dysfluencies are affecting his or her decision-making in education, vocation, and social speaking situations. What activities or situations does he or she avoid because of the dysfluencies (e.g., answering the phone)?

Figures 14.1 and 14.2 provide two interview protocols: one for adults (Figure 14.1) and one for children (Figure 14.2). These protocols provide the clinician with a format for interviewing and exploring the effects of various speaking activities on the rates of dysfluency. As therapy progresses, the stuttering severity inventory provided in Figure 14.3 can be used to record changes in the dysfluency severity.

Task	Time	Total number of responses	Number of dysfluent words	Dysfluent words/minute	Percent fluent
Conversation					
Obtain the case history during this section.	3 min				
Engage the patient in a conversation about his or her speech for 3 min.					
Oral reading					
Have the patient read a 300-word passage aloud.		300 total			
Picture naming					
Have the patient name 10 pictures.		10 total			
Monologue	1 min				
Have the patient speak on any topic for 1 min.					

(To be filled in by therapist unless already filled in)

Task	Time	(To be filled in by therapist unless already filled in)			
		Total number of responses	Number of dysfluent words	Dysfluent words/minute	Percent fluent
Questions					
Ask the patient the following questions:					
"What is your name?"					
"Where do you work?"					
"What exactly do you do there?"					
"What does your father [or husband] do?"					
"What does your mother [or wife] do?"					
"How many are in your family?"					
"Tell me about your family."					
Have the patient ask the examiner five questions.					

Social situation outside the clinician's office				
Accompany the patient as he or she engages a stranger in conversation (e.g., asking for directions).				
Telephone call	1 min			
Have the patient make a 1-min telephone call.				
Total				

Figure 14.1. Dysfluency evaluation for adults. For scoring instructions see the section on dysfluency evaluation. After calculating the totals, make a record of the following: (1) description of type of dysfluencies exhibited, (2) description of secondary or struggle behaviors exhibited, and (3) other observations (e.g., eye contact, facial grimaces, distracting sounds, head movements, or movements of the extremities). (Adapted from BP Ryan. Programmed Therapy for Stuttering in Children and Adults. Springfield, IL: Thomas, 1974;43.)

Task	Time	(To be filled in by therapist unless already filled in)			
		Total number of responses	Number of dysfluent words	Dysfluent words/minute	Percent fluent
Automatic speech tasks					
Have the child count from 1 to 20.		53 total			
Have the child say the alphabet.					
Have the child say the days of the week.					
Imitation		20 total			
Have the child repeat the following: "car," "book," "paper," "yesterday," "happiness," "someday," "See the dog," "That's a good idea," and "Mother and Daddy will come home soon."					
Oral reading		100 total			
Have child read a 100-word passage aloud.					

Picture naming Have the child name 10 pictures.				10 total	
Puppet speech Have child make two puppets talk to each other for 1 min.	1 min				
Monologue Have child speak about any topic for 1 min.	1 min				
Command speech Have the child give the examiner five commands to be performed.					
Have child say nursery rhymes, the alphabet, etc.					
Phonemic difficulty Have the child repeat the following: "vinegar," "cooperation," "linoleum," "spaghetti," "communication," and "socialization."				6 total	

Task	Time	(To be filled in by therapist unless already filled in)			
		Total number of responses	Number of dysfluent words	Dysfluent words/minute	Percent fluent
Speed speech					
Have child name as many items in the room or as many animals as he or she can in 10 sec.					
Questions					
Ask the child the following questions:					
"What does your daddy do?"					
"What does your mother do?"					
"Tell me about your brothers and sisters."					
"Tell me about your pets."					
"Tell me about your favorite show."					
Have the child ask the examiner five questions.					

Conversation							
Engage the child in a conversation about any topic.	3 min						
Speech in another setting							
Observe child in conversation with someone other than the examiner in a setting outside the exam room.	3 min						
Record the location.							
Total							

Figure 14.2. Dysfluency evaluation for preschool and primary age. For scoring instructions see the section on dysfluency evaluation. Omit the items the child cannot perform. After calculating the totals, make a record of the following: (1) description of type of dysfluencies exhibited; (2) description of secondary or struggle behaviors exhibited; and (3) other observations (e.g., eye contact, facial grimaces, distracting sounds, head movements, or movements of the extremities). (Adapted from BP Ryan. Programmed Therapy for Stuttering in Children and Adults. Springfield, IL: Thomas, 1974;34.)

Stuttering Severity Instrument
Glyndon D. Riley, Ph.D.

Name _____ Sex M F Grade _____

School _____ Date of Birth _____

Examiner _____ Date _____ Age _____

I. FREQUENCY

READERS				NONREADERS	
1. Job Task		2. Reading Task			
Percentages	Task Score	Percentages	Task Score	Percentages	Task Score
1	2	1	2	1	4
2-3	3	2-3	4	2-3	6
4	4	4-5	5	4	8
5-6	5	6-9	6	5-6	10
7-9	6	10-16	7	7-9	12
10-14	7	17-26	8	10-14	14
15-28	8	27+	9	15-28	16
29+	9				

Frequency Score: _____ 1 & 2 or 3

II. DURATION

Estimated Length of Three Longest Blocks	Score
Fleeting	1
One half second	2
One full second	3
2 to 9 seconds	4
10 to 30 seconds	5
30 to 60 seconds	6
More than 60 seconds	7

Duration Score: _____

III. PHYSICAL CONCOMITANTS

Evaluating Scale: 0 = none; 1 = not noticeable unless looking for it; 2 = barely noticeable to casual observer; 3 = distracting; 4 = very distracting; 5 = severe and painful looking

Distracting Sounds:	Noisy breathing, whistling, sniffing, blowing, clicking sounds........	0 1 2 3 4 5
Facial Grimaces:	Jaw jerking, tongue protruding, lip pressing, jaw muscles tense....	0 1 2 3 4 5
Head Movements:	Back, forward, turning away, poor eye contact, constant looking around....	0 1 2 3 4 5
Movements of the Extremities:	Arm and hand movement, hands about face, torso movement, leg movements, foot tapping or swinging....	0 1 2 3 4 5

Physical Concomitant Score:
Total Overall Score: _____

Children's Severity Conversion Table				Adult's Severity Conversion Table		
Total Overall Score	Percentile	Severity		Total Overall Score	Percentile	Severity
0-5	0-4	Very Mild		0-16	0-4	Very Mild
6-8	5-11	Mild		17-19	5-11	Mild
9-13	15-23	Mild		20-21	12-23	Mild
14-15	24-40	Mild		22-24	24-40	Moderate
16-19	41-60	Moderate		25-27	41-60	Moderate
20-23	61-77	Moderate		28-30	61-77	Moderate
24-27	78-89	Severe		31-33	78-89	Severe
28-30	90-96	Severe		34-36	90-96	Severe
31-45	97-100	Very Severe		37-45	97-100	Very Severe

Figure 14.3. Stuttering severity instrument. Speakers who can read above a third-grade level are asked to describe their job or school and read a 125-word passage. Nonreaders (anyone who reads below a third-grade level) are shown a cartoon picture and asked to describe what is happening. After this task is complete, engage the patient in conversation. If the dysfluencies are noticeably more severe during **(continued)**

(continued) conversation, use this sample for the frequency count. A total sample of 150 words is required for a frequency count.

Scoring is accomplished across three areas. In the first area, frequency, the first 25 words of the sample are omitted. Count the number of dysfluencies in the next 100 words and convert this to a percentage score. The percentage of dysfluencies is converted to a task score (range of 4–18). In the second area, the duration of the three longest dysfluent moments (fleeting to more than 60 seconds) is tabulated and converted to a task score (range of 1–7). In the third area, physical concomitants across four categories are scaled on a scale of 0 to 5 (0 = none; 5 = severe and painful-looking) and totaled (range of 0–20). The total overall score is calculated by adding the three areas together. The overall score ranges from 0 to 45, which rates the dysfluent behavior from mild to severe. (Reproduced from Riley GD. A stuttering severity instrument for children and adults. J Speech Hear Disord 1972;37:314.)

REFERENCES

1. Manning WH. Clinical Decision Making in the Diagnosis and Treatment of Fluency Disorders. Albany, NY: Delmar Publishers, 1996.
2. Bloodstein O. A Handbook on Stuttering (5th ed). San Diego: Singular, 1995.

SUGGESTED READING

Conture EG. Stuttering (2nd ed). Englewood Cliffs, NJ: Prentice-Hall, 1990.

Nippold MA, Rudzinski M. Parent's speech and children's stuttering: a critique of the literature. J Speech Hear Disord 1995;38:978.

Riley GD. A stuttering severity instrument for children and adults. J Speech Hear Disord 1972;37:314.

Ryan BP. Programmed Therapy for Stuttering in Children and Adults. Springfield, IL: Thomas, 1974.

Van Riper C. The Nature of Stuttering (2nd ed). Englewood Cliffs, NJ: Prentice-Hall, 1982.

Appendix I: National Support Groups and Informational Organizations for People with Speech-Language Disorders

AAC–Augmentative and Alternative Communication
    Journal
c/o Decker Publishing
4 Hughson Street S
P.O. Box 620 LCD1
Hamilton, Ontario L8N 3K7

About Face (international organization for people with
    facial differences)
Box 93
Limekila, PA 19535
(800) 225-FACE
Fax: (610) 689-4479

American Brain Tumor Association (ABTA)
2720 River Road, Suite 146
Des Plaines, IL 60018
(847) 827-9910
(800) 886-2282 (patient services)
Fax: (847) 827-9918

Alcoholics Anonymous
475 Riverside Drive
New York, NY 10115
(212) 870-3400

Alexander Graham Bell Association for the Deaf
3417 Volta Place NW
Washington, DC 20007
(202) 337-5220
Fax: (202) 337-8314

Amyotrophic Lateral Sclerosis Association
21021 Ventura Boulevard, Suite 321
Woodland Hills, CA 91364
(818) 340-2060
(800) 782-4747

Alzheimer's Association
919 North Michigan, Suite 1000
Chicago, IL 60611
(800) 272-3900

American Association for the Education and Rehabilita-
    tion of the Blind and Visually Impaired
206 North Washington Street, Suite 320
Alexandria, VA 22314

American Association of Retired Persons (AARP)
601 E Street NW

Washington, DC 20049
(202) 434-2277
(800) 424-3410

American Cancer Society
1599 Clifton Road NE
Atlanta, GA 30329
(800) ACS-2345

American Council for the Blind
1155 15th NW, Suite 720
Washington, DC 20005
(800) 424-8666

American Diabetes Association
1660 Duke Street
Alexandria, VA 22314
(800) 232-3472

American Foundation for the Blind
15 West 16th Street
New York, NY 10011
(800) AFB-LIND

American Heart Association
7272 Greenville Avenue
Dallas, TX 75231
(214) 373-6300
(800) AHA-USA1

American Lung Association
1740 Broadway
New York, NY 10019
(212) 315-8700

American Parkinson Disease Association
1250 Hylan Boulevard
Staten Island, NY 10305
(800) 223-APDA
Fax: (718) 981-4399

American Society for Deaf Children
2848 Arden Way, Suite 210
Sacramento, CA 95825-1373
(800) 942-ASDC
Fax: (916) 482-0121

American Society on Aging
833 Market Street, Suite 511
San Francisco, CA 94103-1824
(415) 974-9600

American Speech-Language-Hearing Association
10801 Rockville Pike
Rockville, MD 20852-3279
(301) 897-5700
TTY: (301) 897-0157

The ARC (support group for patients with mental retardation and their families)
500 East Border Street, Suite 300
Arlington, TX 76010-7444
(817) 261-6003
Fax: (817) 277-3491

Books on Tape
P.O. Box 7900
Newport Beach, CA 92658
(800) 626-3333

Brain Injury Association
1776 Massachusetts Avenue NW, Suite 100
Washington, DC 20036
(800) 444-6443 (family helpline)
(202) 296-6443

The Brain Tumor Society
84 Seattle Street
Boston, MA 02134
(617) 783-0340
Fax: (617) 783-9712

CAMA-Communications Aids Manufacturers
Association
P.O. Box 1039
Evanston, IL 60204-1039
(800) 441-2262

Fax: (847) 869-5689
E-mail: aac cama@aol.com

Cancer Information Service
(800) 4-CANCER
(800) 422-6237

Cleft Palate Foundation
1218 Grandview Avenue
Pittsburgh, PA 15211
(800) 24-CLEFT
(412) 481-1376
Fax: (412) 481-0847

Foundation for Hospice and Home Care
513 C Street NE
Washington, DC 20002
(202) 547-6586

Guillain-Barré Syndrome Foundation International
P.O. Box 262
Wynnewood, PA 19096
(610) 667-0131
Fax: (610) 667-7036

Huntington's Disease Society of America
140 West 22nd Street, 6th Floor
New York, NY 10011
(212) 242-1968

(800) 345-4372
Fax: (212) 243-2443

International Association for Laryngectomees
(American Cancer Society)
1599 Clifton Road NE
Atlanta, GA 30329
(404) 320-3333

International Fluency Association (IFA)
University of Alabama
Box 870242
Tuscaloosa, AL 35487-0242
(205) 348-7131
Fax: (205) 348-1845
E-mail: ecooper@ua1vm.ua.edu

Multiple Sclerosis Association of America
706 Haddon Field Road
Cherry Hill, NJ 08002
(800) 833-4MSA
Fax: (609) 661-9797

Muscular Dystrophy Association
3300 East Sunrise Drive
Tucson, AZ 85718
(520) 529-2000
Fax: (520) 529-5300

Myasthenia Gravis Foundation
222 South Riverside Plaza, Suite 1540
Chicago, IL 60606
(800) 541-5454
(312) 258-0522
Fax: (312) 258-0461

National Aphasia Association
156 Fifth Avenue
Suite 707
New York, NY 10010
(800) 922-4622

National Association for Homecare
228 7th Street SE
Washington, DC 20003
(202) 547-7424

National Association for the Visually Handicapped
22 West 21st Street, 6th Floor
New York, NY 10010
(212) 889-3141

National Council on Aging
650 South Spring Street, Suite 721
Los Angeles, CA 90014
(213) 622-6151

National Diabetes Information Clearing House
Box NDIC
Bethesda, MD 20205
(301) 496-4000

National Federation of the Blind
1800 Johnson Street
Baltimore, MD 21230
(301) 659-9314

National Library Service for the Blind and Physically
    Handicapped
Library of Congress
1291 Taylor Street NW
Washington, DC 20542
(202) 287-5100

National Multiple Sclerosis Society
3100 Walnut Grove Road
Suite 402
Memphis, TN 38111
(800) 344-4867

Parkinson's Disease Foundation, Inc.
710 W. 168 Street
New York, NY 10032
(212) 923-4700
(800) 457-6676
Fax: (212) 923-4778

Parkinson's Support Groups of America
c/o Ida Raitano
11376 Cherry Hill Road, #204
Beltsville, MD 20705
(301) 937-1545

Rehabilitation Services Administration
Office for the Blind and Visually Impaired
330 C Street SW
Washington, DC 20201
(202) 245-0918

Self Help for the Hard of Hearing (SHHH)
7910 Woodmont Avenue
Suite 1200
Bethesda, MD 20814
(301) 657-2248
Fax: (301) 913-9413
TTY: (301) 657-2249

Stuttering Foundation of America (SFA)
P.O. Box 11749
Memphis, TN 38111-0749
(800) 992-9392
(901) 452-7343
Fax: (901) 452-3931
E-mail: stuttersfa@aol.com

Stuttering Resource Foundation
Ellen Rind Drive
123 Oxford Road
New Rochelle, NY 10804
(800) 232-4773
(914) 632-3925
Fax: (914) 235-0615
E-mail: esr1@inoa.bitnet

United Cerebral Palsy Associations, Inc.
1660 L Street
Suite 700
Washington, DC 20036
(800) 872-5827
Fax: (202) 776-0414

United States Society for Augmentative and Alternative
   Communication (USSAAC)
P.O. Box 5271
Evanston, IL 60204-5271
(847) 869-2122
Fax: (847) 869-2161
E-mail: ussaac@aol.com

Appendix II: Common Prefixes and Suffixes Used in Medical Terminology

Common Medical Prefixes

a(n)-	without, not
ab-	away from, away
ad-	increase, near, toward
ana-	up, increase
ante-	before
anti-	against
bi-	two, both
cata-	down, decrease
con-	together
contra-	opposite, against
cost-	rib
cyst(o)-	sac, bladder
di-	double, two
dia-	through, between
dys-	bad, poor
ecto-	outside
ed-	out of, from
em-, en-	in
end(o)-	within
epi-	upon, in addition
eu-	good, normal
ex-	out

extra-	outside
hemi-	half
hyp(o)-	beneath, deficient
hyper-	above, excessive
iatro-	related to medicine or a physician
inter-	between
intra-	within
leuko-	white
macr(o)-	large
mega-	large
meta-	beyond, change
micro-	small
neutr-	neutral
para-	abnormal, beside, faulty, near
path(o)-	disease, morbid
per-	through, by
peri-	around
poly-	many, much, excessive
pre-	before
pro-	in front of, forward
pseudo-	false
retro-	backward, behind
semi-	half
sub-	below, under
super-, **supra-**	above, beyond, superior
sym-, syn-	with, together, beside
toxi-, toxo-	poisonous
trans-	across

Common Medical Suffixes

-algia	pain
-cele	herniation, protrusion, tumor
-centesis	puncture
-cyte	cell
-dynia	pain
-ectasis	dilatation, expansion
-ectomy	excision
-emesis	vomiting
-emia	blood
-gen, **-genesis**	origination
-genic	caused by, origin
-iasis	condition, formation of
-itis	inflammation
-lysis	breaking down, destruction
-malacia	softening
-megaly	enlargement
-oma	tumor
-opia, **-opsia**	vision
-osis	condition, disease
-path, **-pathy**	disease
-penia	deficiency
-pexy	fixation, suspension
-plasty	surgical correction or repair
-plegia	paralysis

-plexy	fixation
-ptosis	drooping, falling
-ptysis	spitting
-rrhage	gushing, flowing
-rrhaphy	suture
-rrhea	discharge, flow
-scope, -scopy	viewing, inspection
-stalsis	contraction
-stasis	stopped
-staxia	dripping
-stomy	creation of a new opening
-tomy	incision into
-tripsy	crushing
-trophy	development, nourishment

Appendix III: Medical Abbreviations*

Medical abbreviations can have many possible meanings. The context in which they are used should always be considered to ensure proper interpretation. If there is any doubt, ask the attending nurse.

<	less than
>	greater than
A&O	alert and oriented
A&O × 4	alert and oriented to person, place, time, and date
A&O × 3	alert and oriented to person, place, and time
AA	aortic aneurysm; Alcoholics Anonymous
AAA	abdominal aortic aneurysm
AAROM	active assistive range of motion
abd	abductor; abdomen; abdominal
ABG	air/bone gap; arterial blood gases
abnor	abnormal
ACA	adjusted chronologic age; anterior cerebral artery; anterior communicating artery
AD	right ear, admitting diagnosis; Alzheimer's disease

*Information from NM Davis. Medical Abbreviations: 8600 Conveniences at the Expense of Communications and Safety (6th ed). Huntingdon Valley, PA: Neil M. Davis Associates, 1993.

ADD	adduction; attention deficit disorder; average daily dose
ADDH	attention deficit disorder with hyperactivity
ADHD	attention-deficit hyperactivity disorder
ADL	activity of daily living
AER	auditory evoked response; acoustic evoked response
AFib	atrial fibrillation
AGA	appropriate for gestational age; average gestational age
AHHD	arteriosclerotic hypertensive heart disease
AIDS	acquired immune deficiency syndrome
AKA	above-the-knee amputation
ALS	amyotrophic lateral sclerosis; acute lateral sclerosis
AMA	against medical advice; American Medical Association
AMB	ambulation; ambulate
AMI	acute myocardial infarction
AMP	amputation
AODM	adult-onset diabetes mellitus
ARC	acquired immune deficiency syndrome–related complex
ARDS	adult respiratory distress syndrome
ARF	acute renal failure; acute respiratory failure
AROM	active range of motion
AS	left ear; aortic stenosis
ASAP	as soon as possible
ASCVD	arteriosclerotic cardiovascular disease

ASHD	arteriosclerotic heart disease
AU	both ears
AVM	arteriovenous malformation
B&B	bowel and bladder
Ba	barium
BAER	brain stem auditory evoked response
BAL	balance; blood alcohol level
BE	barium enema
BF	black female
bid	twice a day
bilat	bilateral
biw	twice a week
BKA	below-the-knee amputation
BM	bowel movement; black male; bone marrow
BND	bilateral neck dissection
BOT	base of tongue
BP	blood pressure
BPD	bronchopulmonary dysplasia
bpm	beats per minute; breaths per minute
BR	bathroom; bed rest
BT	bowel training; brain tumor; breast tumor
BW	birth weight
Bx	biopsy
c̄	with
c/o	complains of
CA	cancer; cardiac arrest; carotid artery; coronary artery
CABG	coronary artery bypass graft
CAD	coronary artery disease

CBC	complete blood count
CBS	chronic brain syndrome
CC	chief complaint
CCU	critical care unit; coronary care unit; cardiac care unit
CDAP	continuous distended airway pressure
CHF	congestive heart failure
CHI	closed head injury
CIS	carcinoma in situ
CN	cranial nerve
CNS	central nervous system; clinical nurse specialist
cont	continues
coord	coordination
COPD	chronic obstructive pulmonary disease
COTA	certified occupational therapy assistant
CP	cerebral palsy; chest pain; cleft palate
CPAP	continuous positive airway pressure
CPB	cardiopulmonary bypass
CRF	chronic renal failure; chronic respiratory failure
CSF	cerebrospinal fluid
CT or **CAT**	computerized (axial) tomography
CV	cardiovascular
CVA	cardiovascular accident
CVD	cardiovascular disease
CXR	chest x-ray
d/c, DC	discontinue; discharged; decrease

DAT	dementia of Alzheimer's type
DBP	diastolic blood pressure
DF	dorsiflexion
DHT	Dobb-Hoff tube
DJD	degenerative joint disease
DM	diabetes mellitus, diastolic murmur
DM-I	diabetes mellitus type I
DM-II	diabetes mellitus type II
DNR	do not resuscitate
DOB	date of birth
DRG	diagnosis-related group
DVT	deep vein thrombosis
Dx	diagnosis
DZ	disease
ECG	electrocardiogram
ECT	electroconvulsive therapy; emission computed tomography; enhanced computed tomography
EEG	electroencephalogram
EKG or **ECG**	electrocardiogram
EMG	electromyography
EMS	emergency medical system
ENG	electronystagmogram
ENT	ear, nose, throat
ER	emergency room
EST	electroshock therapy
ET	essential tremor; eustachian tube
ET tube	endotracheal tube

ETOH	ethanol
eval	evaluate
EXT	extension; external; extremity
F/U	follow-up
FAS	fetal alcohol syndrome
FD	forceps delivery
FHR	fetal heart rate
FHS	fetal heart sounds
FTT	failure to thrive
FUO	fever of undetermined origin
FVC	forced vital capacity; false vocal cords
FWB	full weight bearing
Fx	fracture
GA	gestational age; general appearance; general anesthesia
GER	gastroesophageal reflux
GI	gastrointestinal
GSW	gunshot wound
H&P	history and physical
H/O	history of
HA	headache; hearing aid; heart attack
HAV	hepatitis A virus
HBO	hyperbaric oxygen
HBP	high blood pressure
HBV	hepatitis B virus; hepatitis B vaccine
HCV	hepatitis C virus
HCVD	hypertensive cardiovascular disease
HEENT	head, eyes, ears, nose, and throat
HEMI	hemiplegia

HH	home health
HI	head injury; hearing impaired
HIV	human immunodeficiency virus
HOH	hard of hearing
HR	heart rate; hospital record; hour
HSV	herpes simplex virus
HTN	hypertension
Hx	history
I&O	intake and output
ICA	internal carotid artery
ICB	intracranial bleed
ICP	intracranial pressure
ICU	intensive care unit; intermediate care unit
IDDM	insulin-dependent diabetes mellitus
IMV	intermittent mandatory ventilation; intermittent mechanical ventilation
IPPB	intermittent positive pressure breathing
IRDM	insulin-resistant diabetes mellitus
IRDS	infant respiratory distress syndrome
IRV	inspiratory reserve volume
IVH	intraventricular hemorrhage
JODM	juvenile-onset diabetes mellitus
L	left; liter; lung; liver
LAT	lateral
LBP	low back pain; low blood pressure
LBW	low birth weight
LE	lower extremity; left ear; left eye
LGA	large for gestational age
LLE	left lower extremity

LOC	loss of consciousness; level of consciousness; level of care
LOS	length of stay
LP	lumbar puncture; light perception
LPN	licensed practical nurse
LT	left; left thigh; light touch
LTG	long-term goal
LTM	long-term memory
LUE	left upper extremity
LUQ	left upper quadrant
max	maximal; maxillary
MCA	middle cerebral artery; middle cerebral aneurysm
MD	muscular dystrophy; medical doctor; manic depression
METS	metastases
MG	myasthenia gravis
MI	myocardial infarction
MIN	minimal
MMR	mumps, measles, and rubella
MOD	moderate
MRI	magnetic resonance imaging
MRSA	methicillin-resistant *Staphylococcus aureus*
MS	multiple sclerosis; mental status; master of science
MSE	mental status examination
MSW	master of social work; multiple stab wounds
MVA	motor vehicle accident
NA	not applicable; Native American

NAD	no acute distress
NDT	neurodevelopmental treatment
NG	nasogastric
NGT	nasogastric tube
NH	nursing home
NICU	neonatal intensive care unit
NIDDM	non–insulin-dependent diabetes mellitus
NKA	no known allergies
NPH	normal pressure hydrocephalus, no previous history
NPO	nothing by mouth (*nil per os*)
NR	no response, no report; normal range; nonreactive
NSG	nursing
N&V	nausea and vomiting
NWB	non–weight-bearing
OA	osteoarthritis
OBS	organic brain syndrome
OD	right eye (oculus dexter); overdose
OM	otitis media
OR	operating room
OS	left eye (oculus sinister); oral surgery
OT	occupational therapy
OU	both eyes (oculi unitas)
p̄	following; after; post
P	pulse
PC	after meals (*post cibus*)
PCA	posterior communicating artery
PEEP	positive end expiratory pressure

PEG	percutaneous endoscopic gastrostomy
PEJ	percutaneous endoscopic jejunostomy
PERL	pupils equal and reactive to light
PERRLA	pupils equal, round, and reactive to light and accommodation
PET	positron emission tomography
PICA	Porch Index of Communicative Ability; posterior inferior cerebellar artery; posterior inferior communicating artery
PMH	past medical history
PMI	past medical illness
PNS	peripheral nervous system
PO	by mouth (*per os*); phone order; post-operative
post-op	postoperative
PPD	packs (of cigarettes) per day
pre-op	before surgery
PRN	as needed (*pro re nata*)
PROM	passive range of motion
PSH	past surgical history
PS	paranoid schizophrenia; physical status; pulmonary stenosis
PT	patient, physical therapy, prothrombin time
PTA	physical therapy assistant; prior to admission
PUD	peptic ulcer disease
PVD	peripheral vascular disease
PWB	partial weight bearing
Px	prognosis; physical exam
q	every

qd	every day
qid	four times a day
quad	quadriplegic
R	right; rate
RA	rheumatoid arthritis; right arm
RAM	rapid alternation movements
RBC	red blood cell; red blood count
RCA	right coronary artery
RDS	respiratory distress syndrome
RDS I	respiratory difficulty due to prematurity
RDS II	respiratory difficulty due to aspiration
rehab	rehabilitation
REPS	repetitions
RH	right hand
RLE	right lower extremity
RLQ	right lower quadrant
R/O	rule out
ROM	range of motion
RT	right; radiation therapy; respiratory therapist; recreational therapy
RUE	right upper extremity
RUQ	right upper quadrant
Rx	treatment; drug; medication; pharmacy; prescription; therapy
$\bar{s}$	without
S/P	status post
SAH	subarachnoid hemorrhage
SCCA	squamous cell carcinoma
SDAT	senile dementia of Alzheimer's type

SGA	small for gestational age
SIDS	sudden infant death syndrome
SNF	skilled nursing facility
SOB	shortness of breath
ST	speech therapy
STD	sexually transmitted disease
STG	short-term goal
STM	short-term memory
Sx	surgery; symptom
syph	syphilis
SZ	seizure; suction; schizophrenic
T	temperature
T&A	tonsillectomy and adenoidectomy
TB	tuberculosis
TBI	traumatic brain injury
TENS	transcutaneous electrical nerve stimulation
THR	total hip replacement
TIA	transient ischemic attack
tid	three times a day
TIS	tumor in situ
TLC	total lung capacity
TM	temperature by mouth; tympanic membrane
TMJ	temporomandibular joint
TNM	tumor, node, metastases
TPR	temperature, pulse, respiration
TURP	transurethral resection of the prostate
Tx	treatment; therapy
UE	upper extremity; undetermined etiology
UGI	upper gastrointestinal series

URI	upper respiratory infection
US	ultrasonography
UTI	urinary tract infection
VD	venereal disease
VF	vision field
VLBW	very low birth weight
VO	verbal order
VSS	vital signs stable
WBC	white blood cell; white blood count
WC	wheelchair
WDWN	well developed and well nourished
WF	white female
WFL	within functional limits; within full limits
WM	white male
WNL	within normal limits
×	times; multiplied by
Y/N	yes/no
YO	years old

Appendix IV: Normal Laboratory Test Values

The values included in this appendix are not for diagnostic purposes, but rather to provide the clinician with additional information. Normal reference values are method dependent and may vary between laboratories.

Laboratory test	Normal value
Hematology	
Activated partial thromboplastin time	25–36 sec
Bleeding time	
Template	2–8 min
Ivy	1–7 min
Duke	1–3 min
Clot retraction	50%
Erythrocyte sedimentation rate	
Males	0–10 mm/hr
Females	0–20 mm/hr
Fibrinogen, plasma	195–365 mg/dl
Fibrin split products	
Screening assay	>10 µg/ml
Quantitative assay	>3 µg/ml
Hematocrit	
Males	42–54%
Females	38–46%
Hemoglobin, total	
Males	14–18 g/dl
Females	12–16 g/dl
Platelet aggregation	3–5 min
Platelet count	130,000–370,000/mm^3

Laboratory test	Normal value
Platelet survival	50% tagged platelets disappear within 84–116 hrs 100% disappear within 8–10 days
Prothrombin consumption time	20 sec
Prothrombin time	
Males	9.6–11.8 sec
Females	9.5–11.3 sec
Red blood cell (RBC) count	
Males	4.5–6.2 million cells/mm^3 venous blood
Females	4.2–5.4 million cells/mm^3 venous blood
Red cell indices	
MCV	84–99 μm^3/red cell
MCH	26–32 pg/red cell
MCHC	30–36%
Reticulocyte count	0.5–2.0% of total RBC count
Sickle cell test	Negative
Thrombin time, plasma	10–15 sec
White blood cell count, blood	4,100–10,900/mm^3
White blood cell differential, blood	
Neutrophils	47.6–76.8%
Lymphocytes	16.2–43.0%
Monocytes	0.6–9.6%
Eosinophils	0.3–7.0%
Basophils	0.3–2.0%
Whole blood clotting time	5–15 min
Blood chemistry	
Acid phosphatase	0.0–1.1 Bodansky units/ml 1–4 King-Armstrong units/ml
Alanine aminotransferase (formerly SGPT)	
Males	10–32 U/liter
Females	9–24 U/liter
Alkaline phosphatase, serum	1.5–4.0 Bodansky units/dl 4.0–13.5 King-Armstrong units/dl

Laboratory test	Normal value
Chemical inhibition method	
Males	90–239 U/dl
Females <45	76–196 U/liter
Females >45	87–250 U/liter
Amylase, serum	60–180 Somogyi units/dl
Arterial blood gases	
PaO_2	75–100 mm Hg
$PaCO_2$	35–45 mm Hg
pH	7.35–7.42
SaO_2	94–100%
HCO_3	22–26 mEq/liter
Aspartate aminotransferase (formerly SGOT)	8–20 U/liter
Bilirubin, serum (adult)	
Direct	<0.5 mg/dl
Indirect	≤1.1 mg/dl
Blood urea nitrogen	8–20 mg/dl
Calcium, serum	4.5–5.5 mEq/liter
Carbon dioxide, total, blood	22–34 mEq/liter
Catecholamines, plasma	
Supine	
Epinephrine	0–110 pg/ml
Norepinephrine	70–750 pg/ml
Dopamine	0–30 pg/ml
Standing	
Epinephrine	0–140 pg/ml
Norepinephrine	200–1700 pg/ml
Dopamine	0–30 pg/ml
Chloride, serum	100–108 mEq/l
Cholesterol, total serum	<200 mg/dl (desirable)
	200–230 mg/dl (borderline range)
C-reactive protein, serum	Negative
Creatine phosphokinase	
Total	
Males	23–99 U/liter
Females	15–57 U/liter

Laboratory test	Normal value
CPK-BB	None
CPK-MB	0–7 IU/liter
CPK-MM	5–70 IU/liter
Creatine, serum	
Males	0.2–0.6 mg/dl
Females	0.6–1.0 mg/dl
Creatinine, serum	
Males	0.8–1.2 mg/dl
Females	0.6–0.9 mg/dl
Free thyroxine	0.8–3.3 ng/dl
Free triiodothyronine	0.2–0.6 ng/dl
Gamma-glutamyltransferase	
Males	6–37 U/liter
Females <age 45	5–27 U/liter
Females >age 45	6–37 U/liter
Glucose, fasting, plasma	70–100 mg/dl
Glucose, plasma, oral tolerance	Peak at 160–180 mg/dl 30–60 min after challenge dose
Glucose, plasma, 2-hour postprandial	<145 mg/dl
Iron, serum	
Males	70–150 µg/dl
Females	80–150 µg/dl
Lactic acid, blood	0.93–1.65 mEq/liter
Lactic dehydrogenase	
Total	48–115 IU/liter
LDH_1	18.1–29%
LDH_2	29.4–37.5%
LDH_3	18.8–26.0%
LDH_4	9.2–16.5%
LDH_5	5.3–13.4%
Lipase	32–80 U/liter
Lipoproteins, serum	
HDL cholesterol	29–77 mg/dl
LDL cholesterol	62–185 mg/dl
Magnesium, serum	1.5–2.5 mEq/liter
Atomic absorption	1.7–2.1 mg/dl

Laboratory test	*Normal value*
Phosphates, serum	1.8–2.6 mEq/liter
Atomic absorption	2.5–4.5 mg/dl
Potassium, serum	3.8–5.5 mEq/liter
Protein, total, serum	6.6–7.9 g/dl
Albumin fraction	3.3–4.5 g/dl
Globulin level	
Alpha globulin	0.1–0.4 g/dl
Alpha$_2$ globulin	0.5–1.0 g/dl
Beta globulin	0.7–1.2 g/dl
Gamma globulin	0.5–1.6 g/dl
Sodium, serum	135–145 mEq/liter
Thyroxine, total, serum	5.0–13.5 µg/dl
Triglycerides, serum	
Ages 0–29	10–140 mg/dl
Ages 30–39	10–150 mg/dl
Ages 40–49	10–160 mg/dl
Ages 50–59	10–190 mg/dl
Uric acid, serum	
Males	4.3–8.0 mg/dl
Females	2.3–6.0 mg/dl
Urine chemistry	
Amylase	10–80 amylase units/hr
Bilirubin	Negative
Calcium	
Males	< 275 mg/24 hrs
Females	< 250 mg/24 hrs
Catecholamines	
24-hour specimen	0–135 µg/dl
Random specimen	0–18 µg/dl
Creatinine	
Males	1.0–1.9 g/24 hrs
Females	0.8–1.7 g/24 hrs
Creatinine clearance	
Males (age 20)	90 ml/min/1.73 m^2
Females (age 20)	84 ml/min/1.73 m^2
Glucose	Negative
17-Hydroxycorticosteroids	

Laboratory test	Normal value
Males	4.5–12.0 mg/24 hrs
Females	2.5–10.0 mg/24 hrs
17-Ketogenic steroids	
Males	4–14 mg/24 hrs
Females	2–12 mg/24 hrs
Ketones	Negative
17-Ketosteroids	
Males	6–21 mg/24 hrs
Females	4–17 mg/24 hrs
Proteins	<150 mg/24 hrs
Sodium	30–280 mEq/24 hrs
Urea	
Maximal clearance	64–99 ml/min
Uric acid	250–750 mg/24 hrs
Urinalysis, routine	
Appearance	Clear
Casts	None, except occasional hyaline casts
Color	Straw
Crystals	Present
Epithelial cells	None
Odor	Slightly aromatic
pH	4.5–8.0
Specific gravity	1.025–1.030
Sugars	None
Yeast cells	None
Urine concentration	
Specific gravity	1.025–1.032
Osmolality	>800 mOsm/kg water
Urine dilution	80% of water excreted in 4 hrs
Specific gravity	<1.003
Osmolality	<100 mOsm/kg water
Urobilinogen	
Males	0.3–2.1 Ehrlich units/2 hrs
Females	0.1–1.1 Ehrlich units/2 hrs
Vanillylmandelic acid	0.7–6.8 mg/24 hrs

Laboratory test	Normal value
Miscellaneous	
Cerebrospinal fluid pressure	50–180 mm H_2O
Enzyme-linked immunosorbent assay (ELISA) for human immunodeficiency virus (HIV) infection	Negative
HIVAGEN test	Negative
Lupus erythematosus cell preparation	Negative
Occult blood, fecal	2.5 mg/24 hrs
Rheumatoid factor, serum	Negative
Urobilinogen, fecal	50–300 mg/24 hrs
Venereal Disease Research Laboratories (VDRL) test, serum	Negative
Western blot assay	Negative

Source: S Loeb (ed). Illustrated Manual of Nursing Practice (2nd ed). Springhouse, PA: Springhouse, 1994;1433.

Appendix V: Pharmacologic Information*

The drugs listed in this appendix are commonly pre-
scribed for anxiety, arthritis, gout, chronic obstructive pulmonary disease (e.g., bronchitis, emphysema, and asthma), depression, hypertension, insomnia, Parkinson's disease, pneumonia, tuberculosis, schizophrenia, transient
ischemic attack, seizures, myasthenia gravis, multiple sclerosis, Gilles de la Tourette's syndrome, and other problems seen in those with speech or language disorders.
This is not an exhaustive list. Some commonly used drugs
have been omitted because they have no adverse reaction
that would have an impact on the speech/language
process. If the drug you are concerned about is not listed
below, do not assume that it does not affect the speech
and language process. If you believe a particular drug
may have an effect on a patient's behavior, seek further
information in the *Physician's Desk Reference* or ask the
patient's physician.

---

*The information in this appendix was taken from D Moreau (ed). Nurs-
ing 96 Drug Handbook. Springhouse, PA: Springhouse, 1996; D Moreau
(ed). Physician's Drug Handbook (6th ed). Springhouse, PA: Springhouse, 1995; and D Vogel, JE Carter. The Effects of Drugs on Communication Disorders. San Diego: Singular, 1995.

Acyclovir

Brand name | Zovirax
Pharmacologic classification | Synthetic purine nucleoside
Therapeutic classification | Antiviral agent
Adverse reactions
    Central nervous system | (Associated with intra-venous dosage) Headache, encephalo-pathic changes (e.g., lethargy, obtundation, tremor, confusion, hallu-cinations, agitation, seizures, coma)

Adrenocorticotropic hormone

Brand names | ACTH, Acthar
Pharmacologic classification | Anterior pituitary hormone
Therapeutic classification | Multiple sclerosis treatment
Adverse reactions
    Central nervous system | Seizures, dizziness, papilledema, headache, euphoria, insomnia, mood swings, personality changes, depression, psychosis

Albuterol

Brand name	Proventil, Proventil Repetabs, Ventolin, Ventolin Rotacaps, Volmax
Pharmacologic classification	Adrenergic
Therapeutic classification	Bronchodilator
Adverse reactions	
Central nervous system	Tremor, nervousness, insomnia, dizziness, headache

Alprazolam

Brand name	Xanax
Pharmacologic classification	Benzodiazepine
Therapeutic classification	Antianxiety agent
Adverse reactions	
Central nervous system	Confusion, drowsiness, light-headedness, headache, hostility, anterograde amnesia, restlessness, psychosis
Eyes, ears, nose, and throat	Visual disturbances
Gastrointestinal system	Dry mouth

Amantadine

Brand names	Symadine, Symmetrel

Pharmacologic classification	Synthetic cyclic primary amine
Therapeutic classification	Antiviral, antiparkinsonian agent
Adverse reactions	
Central nervous system	Depression, fatigue, confusion, dizziness, psychosis, hallucinations, anxiety, irritability, ataxia, insomnia, weakness, headache, light-headedness, difficulty concentrating
Gastrointestinal system	Anorexia, dry mouth

Ambenonium

Brand name	Mytelase
Pharmacologic classification	Cholinesterase inhibitor
Therapeutic classification	Antimyasthenic
Adverse reactions	
Central nervous system	Headache, dizziness, muscle weakness, incoordination, seizures, mental confusion, tremor, nervousness
Eyes, ears, nose, and throat	Miosis
Gastrointestinal system	Increased salivation

Amikacin

Brand names	Amikin
Pharmacologic classification	Aminoglycoside
Therapeutic classification	Antibiotic
Adverse reactions	
Central nervous system	Headache, lethargy, neuro-muscular blockade
Eyes, ears, nose, and throat	Ototoxicity (i.e., tinnitus, vertigo, hearing loss)

Amiloride

Brand name	Midamor
Pharmacologic classification	Potassium-sparing diuretic
Therapeutic classification	Diuretic, antihypertensive
Adverse reactions	
Central nervous system	Dizziness, headache, weakness
Gastrointestinal system	Anorexia

Amitriptyline

Brand name	Elavil, Emitrip, Endep, Enovil, PMS-Amitriptyline
Pharmacologic classification	Tricyclic antidepressant
Therapeutic classification	Antidepressant

Adverse reactions

Central nervous system	Drowsiness, dizziness, excitation, tremors, weakness, confusion, headache, nervousness, electroencephalographic (EEG) changes, seizures, extrapyramidal reactions
Eyes, ears, nose, and throat	Blurred vision, tinnitus
Gastrointestinal system	Dry mouth, anorexia

Amobarbital

Brand name	Amytal, Amytal Sodium
Pharmacologic classification	Barbiturate
Therapeutic classification	Sedative-hypnotic, anti-hypnotic

Adverse reactions

Central nervous system	Drowsiness, lethargy, hangover, paradoxical excitement

Anistreplase

Brand name	Eminase
Pharmacologic classification	Thrombolytic enzyme
Therapeutic classification	Thrombolytic enzyme
Adverse reactions	
Central nervous system	Intracranial hemorrhage
Eyes, ears, nose, and throat	Gum or mouth hemorrhage

Atenolol

Brand name	Tenormin
Pharmacologic classification	Beta-adrenergic blocking agent
Therapeutic classification	Antihypertensive, antianginal
Adverse reactions	
Central nervous system	Fatigue, lethargy

Aurothioglucose

Brand name	Solganal
Pharmacologic classification	Gold salt
Therapeutic classification	Antiarthritic
Adverse reactions	
Central nervous system	Dizziness, syncope
Gastrointestinal system	Difficulty swallowing

Baclofen

Brand name	Lioresal, Lioresal Intra-thecal
Pharmacologic classification	Chlorophenol derivative
Therapeutic classification	Skeletal muscle relaxant
Adverse reactions	
Central nervous system	Drowsiness, dizziness, headache, weakness, fatigue, confusion, insomnia, dysarthria, seizures
Eyes, ears, nose, and throat	Blurred vision

Benazepril

Brand name	Lotensin
Pharmacologic classification	Angiotensin-converting enzyme (ACE) inhibitor
Therapeutic classification	Antihypertensive
Adverse reactions	
Central nervous system	Headache, dizziness, light-headedness, anxiety, amnesia, depression, insomnia, nervousness, neuralgia, neuropathy, paresthesia, somnolence
Eyes, ears, nose, and throat	Dysphagia, increased salivation
Gastrointestinal system	Dry, persistent, nonproductive cough

Benztropine

Brand names	Cogentin
Pharmacologic classification	Anticholinergic
Therapeutic classification	Antiparkinsonian agent
Adverse reactions	
Central nervous system	Disorientation, restlessness, irritability, incoherence, hallucinations, headache, sedation, depression, muscular weakness

Eyes, ears, nose, and throat	Dilated pupils, blurred vision, photophobia, difficulty swallowing
Gastrointestinal system	Dry mouth

Betaxolol

Brand names	Betoptic
Pharmacologic classification	Beta-adrenergic blocking agent
Therapeutic classification	Antiglaucoma agent, antihypertensive
Adverse reactions	
Central nervous system	Insomnia, confusion

Biperiden

Brand names	Akineton, Akineton Lactate
Pharmacologic classification	Anticholinergic
Therapeutic classification	Antiparkinsonian agent
Adverse reactions	
Central nervous system	Disorientation, euphoria, restlessness, irritability, incoherence, dizziness, increased tremor
Eyes, ears, nose, and throat	Blurred vision
Gastrointestinal system	Dry mouth

Bisoprolol

Brand names	Zebeta
Pharmacologic classification	Beta-adrenergic blocking agent
Therapeutic classification	Antihypertensive
Adverse reactions	
Central nervous system	Asthenia, dizziness, fatigue, headache, hypoesthesia, vivid dreams, depression, insomnia
Gastrointestinal system	Dry mouth
Respiratory system	Cough, dyspnea

Bromocriptine

Brand name	Parlodel
Pharmacologic classification	Dopamine-receptor agonist
Therapeutic classification	Semisynthetic ergot alkaloid; dopaminergic agonist; antiparkinsonian agent
Adverse reactions	
Central nervous system	Confusion, hallucination, uncontrolled body movements, dizziness, headache, fatigue, mania, delusions, nervousness, insomnia, depression, seizures

| Eyes, ears, nose, and throat | Tinnitus, blurred vision |
| Respiratory system | Pulmonary infiltration and pleural effusion |

Bumetanide

Brand name	Bumex
Pharmacologic classification	Loop diuretic
Therapeutic classification	Diuretic
Adverse reactions	
Central nervous system	Dizziness, headache
Eyes, ears, nose, and throat	Transient deafness

Bupropion

Brand name	Wellbutrin
Pharmacologic classification	Aminoketone
Therapeutic classification	Antidepressant
Adverse reactions	
Central nervous system	Headache, akathisia, seizures, agitation, anxiety, confusion, delusions, euphoria, hostility, impaired sleep quality, insomnia, sedation, sensory disturbance, tremor
Eyes, ears, nose, and throat	Auditory disturbances, blurred vision
Gastrointestinal system	Dry mouth, taste disturbance

Butabarbital

Brand name	Butalan, Butisol, Sarisol No. 2
Pharmacologic classification	Barbiturate
Therapeutic classification	Sedative-hypnotic
Adverse reactions	
Central nervous system	Drowsiness, lethargy, hangover, paradoxic excitement in elderly patients
Respiratory system	Respiratory depression

Captopril

Brand name	Capoten
Pharmacologic classification	ACE inhibitor
Therapeutic classification	Antihypertensive, adjunctive treatment of congestive heart failure
Adverse reactions	
Central nervous system	Dizziness, fainting
Gastrointestinal system	Anorexia, dysgeusia (loss of taste)
Respiratory system	Dry, persistent, nonproductive cough

Carbamazepine

Brand names	Epitol, Tegretol

Pharmacologic classification	Iminostilbene derivative; chemically related to tricyclic antidepressants
Therapeutic classification	Anticonvulsant, analgesic

Adverse reactions

Central nervous system	Dizziness, vertigo, drowsiness, fatigue, ataxia, worsening of seizures (usually in patients with mixed seizure disorders)
Eyes, ears, nose, and throat	Conjunctivitis, dry mouth and pharynx, blurred vision, diplopia, nystagmus
Gastrointestinal system	Anorexia

Carbidopa-levodopa

Brand names	Sinemet, Sinemet CR
Pharmacologic classification	Decarboxylase inhibitor–dopamine precursor combination
Therapeutic classification	Antiparkinsonian agent

Adverse reactions

Central nervous system	Choreiform movements, dystonic and dyskinetic movements, involuntary grimacing, head movements, myoclonic body

	jerks, ataxia, tremors, muscle twitching, brady-kinetic episodes, psychiatric disturbances, memory loss, nervousness, anxiety, disturbing dreams, euphoria, malaise, fatigue, severe depression, suicidal tendencies, dementia, delirium, hallucinations
Eyes, ears, nose, and throat	Blurred vision, diplopia, excessive salivation
Gastrointestinal system	Dry mouth, bitter taste, anorexia

Carteolol

Brand names	Cartrol
Pharmacologic classification	Beta-adrenergic blocking agent
Therapeutic classification	Antihypertensive
Adverse reactions	
Central nervous system	Lassitude, tiredness, fatigue, somnolence, asthenia

Cephalexin

| Brand names | Keftab, Cefanex, C-Lexin, Keflet, Keflex |

Pharmacologic classification	First-generation cephalosporin
Therapeutic classification	Antibiotic
Adverse reactions	
Central nervous system	Dizziness, headache, malaise, paresthesias, seizures
Gastrointestinal system	Anorexia, oral candidiasis

Cephalothin

Brand names	Keflin
Pharmacologic classification	First-generation cephalosporin
Therapeutic classification	Antibiotic
Adverse reactions	
Central nervous system	Dizziness, headache, malaise, paresthesias
Gastrointestinal system	Anorexia, oral candidiasis

Chlordiazepoxide

Brand name	Libritabs, Librium, Lipoxide
Pharmacologic classification	Benzodiazepine
Therapeutic classification	Antianxiety agent, anticonvulsant, sedative-hypnotic
Adverse reactions	
Central nervous system	Drowsiness, lethargy, hangover, fainting, restless-

	ness, psychosis, suicidal tendencies
Eyes, ears, nose, and throat	Visual disturbances

Chlorpromazine

Brand name	Ormazine, Thorazine, Thor-Prom
Pharmacologic classification	Aliphatic phenothiazine
Therapeutic classification	Antipsychotic
Adverse reactions	
Central nervous system	Extrapyramidal reactions, sedation, tardive dyskinesia, pseudoparkinsonism, dizziness
Eyes, ears, nose, and throat	Blurred vision
Gastrointestinal system	Dry mouth

Ciprofloxacin

Brand name	Cipro, Cipro I.V.
Pharmacologic classification	Fluoroquinolone antibiotic
Therapeutic classification	Antibiotic
Adverse reactions	
Central nervous system	Headache, restlessness, tremor, light-headedness, confusion, hallucinations, seizures, paresthesia
Gastrointestinal system	Nausea, vomiting, oral candidiasis

Clomipramine

Brand name	Anafranil
Pharmacologic classification	Tricyclic antidepressant
Therapeutic classification	Antiobsessional agent
Adverse reactions	
Central nervous system	Somnolence, tremors, dizziness, headache, insomnia, nervousness, myoclonus, fatigue, EEG changes, seizures, extrapyramidal reactions, asthenia, aggressiveness
Eyes, ears, nose, and throat	Otitis media (in children), abnormal vision, laryngitis, pharyngitis
Gastrointestinal system	Dry mouth, anorexia

Clonazepam

Brand names	Klonopin
Pharmacologic classification	Benzodiazepine
Therapeutic classification	Anticonvulsant
Adverse reactions	
Central nervous system	Drowsiness, ataxia, behavioral disturbances (especially in children), slurred speech, tremor, confusion, psychosis, agitation

Eyes, ears, nose, and throat	Increased salivation, diplopia, nystagmus, abnormal eye movements, sore gums
Respiratory system	Respiratory depression

Clonidine

Brand name	Catapres, Catapres-TTS
Pharmacologic classification	Ventrally acting antiadrenergic agent
Therapeutic classification	Antihypertensive
Adverse reactions	
Central nervous system	Drowsiness, dizziness, fatigue, sedation, nervousness, headache, vivid dreams
Gastrointestinal system	Dry mouth

Clorazepate

Brand names	Gen-XENE, Tranxene, Tranxene-SD, Tranxene-T-Tab
Pharmacologic classification	Benzodiazepine
Therapeutic classification	Antianxiety agent, anticonvulsant, sedative-hypnotic

Adverse reactions
    Central nervous system

Drowsiness, lethargy, hangover, fainting, restlessness, psychosis

    Eyes, ears, nose, and throat   Visual disturbances
    Gastrointestinal system   Dry mouth

Clozapine

Brand name   Clozaril
Pharmacologic classification Tricyclic dibenzodiazepine derivative

Therapeutic classification   Antipsychotic
Adverse reactions
    Central nervous system

Drowsiness, sedation, seizures, dizziness, syncope, vertigo, headache, tremor, disturbed sleep or nightmares, restlessness, hyperkinesia, hypokinesia, akinesia, agitation, rigidity, akathisia, confusion, fatigue, insomnia, weakness, lethargy, ataxia, slurred speech, depression, myoclonus, anxiety

    Gastrointestinal system

Dry mouth, excessive salivation

Cyclosporine

Brand names	Sandimmune
Pharmacologic classification	Polypeptide antibiotic
Therapeutic classification	Immunosuppressant
Adverse reactions	
Central nervous system	Tremor, headache
Eyes, ears, nose, and throat	Oral thrush

Dantrolene

Brand names	Dantrium, Dantrium Intravenous
Pharmacologic classification	Hydantoin derivative
Therapeutic classification	Skeletal muscle relaxant
Adverse reactions	
Central nervous system	Muscle weakness, drowsiness, dizziness, lightheadedness, malaise, headache, confusion, nervousness, insomnia, hallucinations, seizures
Eyes, ears, nose, and throat	Auditory or visual disturbances
Gastrointestinal system	Anorexia, dysphagia

Desipramine

Brand name	Norpramin, Pertofrane

Pharmacologic classification	Dibenzazepine tricyclic antidepressant
Therapeutic classification	Antidepressant, antianxiety agent

Adverse reactions
    Central nervous system — Drowsiness, dizziness, excitation, tremors, weakness, confusion, headache, nervousness, EEG changes, seizures, extrapyramidal reactions

    Eyes, ears, nose, and throat — Blurred vision, tinnitus

    Gastrointestinal system — Dry mouth, anorexia

Dexamethasone

Brand name — Decadron, Dexamethasone Intensol, Dexone 0.5, Dexone 0.75, Dexone 1.5, Dexone 4, Hexadrol, Mymethasone, Dalalone D.P., Dalalone L.A., Decadron-LA, Decaject-L.A., Dexacen LA-8, Dexasone-LA, Dexone LA, Solurex-LA, Ak-Dex, Dalalone, Decadrol, Decadron Phosphate, Decaject, Dexacen-4,

	Dexone, Hexadrol Phosphate, Solurex
Pharmacologic classification	Glucocorticoid
Therapeutic classification	Anti-inflammatory, immunosuppressant
Adverse reactions	
Central nervous system	Euphoria, insomnia, psychotic behavior, pseudotumor cerebri

Dextroamphetamine

Brand names	Dexedrine, Dexedrine Spansule, Oxydess II, Robese, Spancap #1
Pharmacologic classification	Amphetamine
Therapeutic classification	Central nervous system stimulant, short-term adjunctive anorexigenic agent, sympathomimetic amine
Adverse reactions	
Central nervous system	Restlessness, tremor, insomnia, dizziness, headache, chills, overstimulation, dysphoria
Gastrointestinal system	Dry mouth, anorexia

Diazepam

Brand names	Diazepam Intensol, T-Quil, Valium, Valrelease, Vazepam, Zetran
Pharmacologic classification	Benzodiazepine
Therapeutic classification	Anticonvulsant, antianxiety agent, sedative-hypnotic

Adverse reactions

Central nervous system	Drowsiness, lethargy, hangover, ataxia, fainting, depression, restlessness, anterograde amnesia, psychosis, slurred speech, tremor
Eyes, ears, nose, and throat	Diplopia, blurred vision, nystagmus
Respiratory system	Respiratory depression

Dicloxacillin

Brand names	Dycill, Dynapen, Pathocil
Pharmacologic classification	Penicillinase-resistant penicillin
Therapeutic classification	Antibiotic

Adverse reactions

Central nervous system	Neuromuscular irritability, seizures

Digitoxin

Brand name	Crystodigin
Pharmacologic classification	Digitalis
Therapeutic classification	Antiarrhythmic, inotropic
Adverse reactions	
Central nervous system	Fatigue, generalized weakness, agitation, hallucinations, headache, malaise, dizziness, vertigo, stupor, paresthesias
Eyes, ears, nose, and throat	Diplopia, blurred vision, photophobia

Digoxin

Brand names	Digoxin, Lanoxicaps, Lanoxin
Pharmacologic classification	Digitalis
Therapeutic classification	Antiarrhythmic, inotropic
Adverse reactions	
Central nervous system	Fatigue, generalized weakness, agitation, hallucinations, headache, malaise, dizziness, vertigo, stupor, paresthesias
Eyes, ears, nose, and throat	Diplopia, blurred vision, photophobia
Gastrointestinal system	Anorexia

Diltiazem

Brand name	Cardizem, Cardizem CD, Cardizem SR, Dilacor XR
Pharmacologic classification	Calcium channel blocker
Therapeutic classification	Antianginal
Adverse reactions	
Central nervous system	Headache, fatigue, drowsiness, dizziness, nervousness, depression, insomnia, confusion

Doxepin

Brand name	Adapin, Sinequan
Pharmacologic classification	Tricyclic antidepressant
Therapeutic classifcation	Antidepressant
Adverse reactions	
Central nervous system	Drowsiness, dizziness, excitation, tremors, weakness, confusion, headache, nervousness, EEG changes, seizures, extrapyramidal reactions
Eyes, ears, nose, and throat	Blurred vision, tinnitus
Gastrointestinal system	Dry mouth, anorexia

Edrophonium

Brand names	Enlon, Reversol, Tensilon
Pharmacologic classification	Cholinesterase inhibitor
Therapeutic classification	Cholinergic agonist, diagnostic agent
Adverse reactions	
Central nervous system	Seizures, weakness, dysarthria, dysphagia, sweating
Eyes, ears, nose, and throat	Diplopia, miosis, conjunctival hyperemia
Gastrointestinal system	Excessive salivation

Enalaprilat

Enalapril maleate

Brand names	Vasotec I.V. (enalaprilat) Vasotec (enalapril maleate)
Pharmacologic classification	ACE inhibitor
Therapeutic classification	Antihypertensive
Adverse reactions	
Central nervous system	Headache, dizziness, lightheadedness, fatigue, insomnia
Respiratory system	Dry, persistent, nonproductive cough

Epinephrine

Brand name	Adrenalin, Bronkaid Mist, Primatene Mist, Asthma-Haler, Bronitin Mist, Bronkaid Mist Suspension, Medihaler-Epi, Primatene Mist Suspension, Adrenalin Chloride, Epi-Pen, Epi-Pen Jr., Sus-Phrine
Pharmacologic classification	Adrenergic
Therapeutic classification	Bronchodilator, vasopressor, cardiac stimulant, local anesthetic, topical antihemorrhagic, antiglaucoma agent
Adverse reactions	
Central nervous system	Nervousness, tremor, euphoria, anxiety, coldness of extremities, vertigo, headache, diaphoresis, disorientation, agitation, increase of rigidity and tremor in patients with Parkinson's disease.

Erythromycin

Brand names	Ilotycin, Erythrocin

Pharmacologic classification	Erythromycin
Therapeutic classification	Antibiotic
Adverse reactions	
Eyes, ears, nose, and throat	Hearing loss with high intravenous doses

Estazolam

Brand name	ProSom
Pharmacologic classification	Benzodiazepine
Therapeutic classification	Antianxiety agent
Adverse reactions	
Central nervous system	Fatigue, dizziness, daytime drowsiness, somnolence, asthenia, hypokinesia, headache

Ethacrynate

Ethacrynic acid

Brand names	Sodium Edecrin (ethacrynate) Edecrin (ethacrynic acid)
Pharmacologic classification	Loop diuretic
Therapeutic classification	Diuretic
Adverse reactions	
Eyes, ears, nose, and throat	Transient deafness with too rapid intravenous injection

Ethotoin

Brand name	Peganone
Pharmacologic classification	Hydantoin derivative
Therapeutic classification	Anticonvulsant
Adverse reactions	
Central nervous system	Fatigue, insomnia, dizziness, headache, numbness, slurred speech, ataxia
Eyes, ears, nose, and throat	Diplopia, nystagmus

Felbamate

Brand name	Felbatol
Pharmacologic classification	Dicarbamate anticonvulsant
Therapeutic classification	Anticonvulsant
Adverse reactions	
Central nervous system	Headache, insomnia, fatigue, anxiety
Eyes, ears, nose, and throat	Blurred or double vision, otitis media

Felodipine

Brand name	Plendil
Pharmacologic classification	Calcium channel blocker
Therapeutic classification	Antihypertensive
Adverse reactions	
Central nervous system	Headache, dizziness, paresthesia, asthenia

Respiratory system	Upper respiratory infection, cough

Fluoxetine

Brand name	Prozac
Pharmacologic classification	Serotonin uptake inhibitor
Therapeutic classification	Antidepressant
Adverse reactions	
Central nervous system	Headache, nervousness, insomnia, drowsiness, anxiety, tremor, dizziness, asthenia, abnormal dreams
Eyes, ears, nose, and throat	Cough, visual disturbances, tinnitus
Gastrointestinal system	Nausea, dry mouth, anorexia, taste change
Respiratory system	Upper respiratory infection, respiratory distress

Fluphenazine

Brand name	Permitil, Permitil Concentrate, Prolixin, Prolixin Oral Concentrate
Pharmacologic classification	Phenothiazine (piperazine derivative)
Therapeutic classification	Antipsychotic

Adverse reactions
    Central nervous system   Extrapyramidal reactions,
                                              tardive dyskinesia,
                                              sedation, pseudoparkin-
                                              sonism, EEG changes,
                                              dizziness
    Eyes, ears, nose, and throat   Blurred vision
    Gastrointestinal system   Dry mouth

Flurazepam

Brand name   Dalmane
Pharmacologic classification   Benzodiazepine
Therapeutic classification   Sedative-hypnotic
Adverse reactions
    Central nervous system   Confusion, drowsiness,
                                              lethargy, daytime seda-
                                              tion, disturbed coordina-
                                              tion, dizziness, headache

Fosinopril

Brand name   Monopril
Pharmacologic classification   ACE inhibitor
Therapeutic classification   Antihypertensive
Adverse reactions
    Central nervous system   Headache, dizziness,
                                              fatigue, light-headedness,
                                              syncope, memory distur-
                                              bances, mood changes,

paresthesia, sleep disturbance, drowsiness, weakness, cerebrovascular accidents

Eyes, ears, nose, and throat	Tinnitus, vision disturbances, eye irritation
Gastrointestinal system	Dysphagia, dry mouth
Respiratory system	Dry, persistent, nonproductive cough, laryngitis, hoarseness

Furosemide

Brand name	Lasix, Myrosemide
Pharmacologic classification	Loop diuretic
Therapeutic classification	Diuretic, antihypertensive
Adverse reactions	
Eyes, ears, nose, and throat	Transient deafness with too rapid intravenous injection

Gabapentin

Brand names	Neurontin
Pharmacologic classification	Aminoglycoside
Therapeutic classification	Anticonvulsant
Adverse reactions	
Central nervous system	Somnolence, dizziness, ataxia, fatigue, nystagmus,

| | tremor, nervousness, dysarthria, amnesia, depression, abnormal thinking, twitching, abnormal coordination |
| Eyes, ears, nose, and throat | Diplopia, dry mouth and throat, coughing |

Gentamicin

Brand names	Garamycin, Gentamicin Sulfate ADD-Vantage, Jenamicin
Pharmacologic classification	Aminoglycoside
Therapeutic classification	Antibiotic
Adverse reactions	
Central nervous system	Headache, lethargy, neuro-muscular blockade
Eyes, ears, nose, and throat	Ototoxicity (i.e., tinnitus, vertigo, hearing loss)

Gold sodium thiomalate

Brand name	Myochrysine
Pharmacologic classification	Gold salt
Therapeutic classification	Antiarthritic
Adverse reactions	
Central nervous system	Dizziness, syncope
Gastrointestinal system	Difficulty swallowing

Guanadrel

Brand name	Hylorel
Pharmacologic classification	Adrenergic neuron blocking agent
Therapeutic classification	Antihypertensive
Adverse reactions	
Central nervous system	Fatigue, dizziness, drowsiness, faintness
Gastrointestinal system	Dry mouth

Guanethidine

Brand name	Ismelin
Pharmacologic classification	Adrenergic neuron blocking agent
Therapeutic classification	Antihypertensive
Adverse reactions	
Central nervous system	Dizziness, weakness, syncope
Gastrointestinal system	Dry mouth

Haloperidol

Brand name	Haldol, Halperon
Pharmacologic classification	Butyrophenone
Therapeutic classification	Antipsychotic
Adverse reactions	
Central nervous system	Severe extrapyramidal reactions, tardive dyskinesia, sedation

Eyes, ears, nose, and throat   Blurred vision

Hydralazine

Brand name   Apresoline
Pharmacologic classification   Peripheral vasodilator
Therapeutic classification   Antihypertensive
Adverse reactions
    Central nervous system   Peripheral neuritis,
        headache, dizziness

    Gastrointestinal system   Anorexia

Hydroxyzine

Brand name   Anxanil, Atarax, Atozine,
    Durrax, E-Vista, Hydrox-
    acen, Hyzine-50, Quiess,
    Vistacon-50, Vistaject-25,
    Vistaject-50, Vistaquel,
    Vistaril, Vistazine-50, Hy-
    Pam, Vamate, Vistaril
Pharmacologic classification   Antihistamine
Therapeutic classification   Antianxiety agent, sedative,
    antipruritic, antiemetic,
    antispasmodic
Adverse reactions
    Central nervous system   Drowsiness, ataxia, involun-
        tary motor activity
    Eyes, ears, nose, and throat Dry mouth

Ibuprofen

Brand name	Aches-N-Pain, Advil, Children's Advil, Excedrin-IB Caplets, Excedrin-IB Tablets, Genpril Caplets, Genpril Tablets, Haltran, Ibuprin, Ibuprohm Caplets, Ibuprohm Tablets, Ibu-Tab, Medipren Caplets, Midol-200, Motrin, Motrin IB Caplets, Nuprin Caplets, Nuprin Tablets, Pamprin-IB, PediaProfen, Rufen, Saleto-200, Saleto-400, Saleto-600, Saleto-800, Trendar
Pharmacologic classification	Nonsteroidal anti-inflammatory
Therapeutic classification	Non-narcotic analgesic, antipyretic, anti-inflammatory
Adverse reactions	
Central nervous system	Headache, drowsiness, dizziness, aseptic meningitis, cognitive dysfunction
Eyes, ears, nose, and throat	Vision disturbances, tinnitus

Imipramine

Brand name	Janimine, Norfranil, Tipramine, Tofranil, Tofranil-PM
Pharmacologic classification	Dibenzazepine tricyclic antidepressant
Therapeutic classification	Antidepressant, antianxiety agent
Adverse reactions	
Central nervous system	Drowsiness, dizziness, excitation, tremors, weakness, headache, nervousness, seizures, extrapyramidal symptoms, confusion, EEG changes
Eyes, ears, nose, and throat	Blurred vision, tinnitus
Gastrointestinal system	Dry mouth, anorexia

Indapamide

Brand name	Lozol
Pharmacologic classification	Thiazide-like diuretic
Therapeutic classification	Diuretic, antihypertensive
Adverse reactions	
Central nervous system	Headache, irritability, nervousness, dizziness, lightheadedness, weakness
Gastrointestinal system	Anorexia

Indomethacin

Brand name	Indameth, Indochron E-R, Indocin, Indocin SR, Indocin IV
Pharmacologic classification	Nonsteroidal anti-inflammatory
Therapeutic classification	Non-narcotic analgesic, antipyretic, anti-inflammatory
Adverse reactions	
Central nervous system	Headache, drowsiness, dizziness, depression, confusion, peripheral neuropathy, seizures, psychic disturbances, syncope, vertigo
Eyes, ears, nose, and throat	Blurred vision, corneal and retinal damage, hearing loss, tinnitus
Gastrointestinal system	Anorexia

Interferon beta-1b

Brand name	Betaseron
Pharmacologic classification	Biological response modifier
Therapeutic classification	Antiviral, immunoregulator
Adverse reactions	
Central nervous system	Depression, anxiety, emotional lability, deperson-

| | alization, suicidal tendencies, confusion, somnolence, headache, dizziness |
| Eyes, ears, nose, and throat | Laryngitis |

Isocarboxazid

Brand name	Marplan
Pharmacologic classification	Monoamine oxidase inhibitor
Therapeutic classification	Antidepressant
Adverse reactions	
Central nervous system	Dizziness, vertigo, weakness, headache, hyperactivity, hyperreflexia, tremors, muscle twitching, mania, insomnia, confusion, memory impairment, fatigue
Eyes, ears, nose, and throat	Blurred vision
Gastrointestinal system	Dry mouth, anorexia, nausea

Isoproterenol

| Brand name | Aerolone, Day-Dose Isoproterenol, Dispos-a-Med Isoproterenol, Isuprel, Vapo-Iso, Isuprel Glossets, Isuprel Mis- |

	tometer, Norisodrine Aerotrol, Medihaler-Iso
Pharmacologic classification	Adrenergic
Therapeutic classification	Bronchodilator, cardiac stimulant
Adverse reactions	
Central nervous system	Nervousness, insomnia, weakness, dizziness, mild tremor, headache

Isosorbide

Brand name	Dilatrate-SR, Iso-Bid, Isonate, Isorbid, Isordil, Isotrate, Sorbitrate, Sorbitrate Sustained Action, Imdur, Ismo, Monoket
Pharmacologic classification	Nitrate
Therapeutic classification	Antianginal agent
Adverse reactions	
Central nervous system	Dizziness, headache, weakness

Isradipine

Brand name	DynaCirc
Pharmacologic classification	Calcium channel blocker
Therapeutic classification	Antihypertensive
Adverse reactions	
Central nervous system	Dizziness

Kanamycin

Brand names	Kantrex
Pharmacologic classification	Aminoglycoside
Therapeutic classification	Antibiotic
Adverse reactions	
Central nervous system	Headache, lethargy, neuro-muscular blockade
Eyes, ears, nose, and throat	Ototoxicity (i.e., tinnitus, vertigo, hearing loss)

Levodopa (L-dopa)

Brand names	Dopar, Larodopa
Pharmacologic classification	Precursor of dopamine
Therapeutic classification	Antiparkinsonian agent
Adverse reaction	
Central nervous system	Aggressive behavior, choreiform movements, dystonic and dyskinetic movements, involuntary grimacing, head movements, myoclonic body jerks, ataxia, tremors, muscle twitching, bradykinetic episodes, psychiatric disturbances, memory loss, mood changes, nervousness, anxiety, disturbing dreams, eupho-

	ria, malaise, fatigue, severe depression, suicidal tendencies, dementia, delirium, hallucinations
Eyes, ears, nose, and throat	Blurred vision, diplopia, excessive salivation
Gastrointestinal system	Dry mouth, bitter taste, anorexia

Lisinopril

Brand name	Prinivil, Zestril
Pharmacologic classification	ACE inhibitor
Therapeutic classification	Antihypertensive
Adverse reactions	
Central nervous system	Headache, dizziness, fatigue, depression, somnolence, paresthesia
Gastrointestinal system	Dry, persistent, nonproductive cough

Lithium

Brand name	Eskalith, Eskalith CR, Lithobid, Lithonate, Lithotabs
Pharmacologic classification	Alkali metal
Therapeutic classification	Antimanic, antipsychotic
Adverse reactions	

Central nervous system	Tremors, drowsiness, headache, confusion, restlessness, dizziness, psychomotor retardation, stupor, lethargy, coma, blackouts, epileptiform seizures, EEG changes, worsened organic mental syndrome, impaired speech, ataxia, muscle weakness, incoordination
Eyes, ears, nose, and throat	Tinnitus, blurred vision
Gastrointestinal system	Dry mouth, nausea, anorexia

Lorazepam

Brand names	Alzapam, Ativan, Lorazepam Intensol
Pharmacologic classification	Antianxiety agent
Therapeutic classification	Anticonvulsant
Adverse reactions	
Central nervous system	Drowsiness, lethargy, hangover, fainting, anterograde amnesia, restlessness, psychosis
Eyes, ears, nose, and throat	Vision disturbances
Gastrointestinal system	Dry mouth

Loxapine

Brand name	Loxitane C, Loxitane IM, Loxitane
Pharmacologic classification	Dibenzoxazepine
Therapeutic classification	Antipsychotic
Adverse reactions	
Central nervous system	Extrapyramidal reactions, sedation, tardive dyskinesia, pseudoparkinsonism, EEG changes, dizziness
Eyes, ears, nose, and throat	Blurred vision
Gastrointestinal system	Dry mouth

Mannitol

Brand names	Osmitrol
Pharmacologic classification	Osmotic diuretic
Therapeutic classification	Diuretic (prevention and management of acute renal failure or oliguria, reduction of intracranial or intraocular pressure, treatment of drug intoxication)
Adverse reactions	
Central nervous system	Rebound increase in intracranial pressure

8–12 hours after diuresis,
headache, confusion

Eyes, ears, nose, and throat   Blurred vision

Mephenytoin

Brand names   Mesantoin
Pharmacologic classification   Hydantoin derivative
Therapeutic classification   Anticonvulsant
Adverse reactions
    Central nervous system   Drowsiness, ataxia, fatigue,
irritability, choreiform
movements, depression,
tremor, sleeplessness,
dizziness

Eyes, ears, nose, and throat   Diplopia, nystagmus

Meprobamate

Brand names   Equanil, Meprospan-200,
Meprospan-400, Mil-
town-200, Miltown-400,
Miltown-600, Probate,
Trancot
Pharmacologic classification   Carbamate
Therapeutic classification   Antianxiety agent
Adverse reactions
    Central nervous system   Dizziness, drowsiness,
ataxia, slurred speech,

| | headache, vertigo, seizures |
| Gastrointestinal system | Anorexia |

Methyldopa

Brand name	Aldomet
Pharmacologic classification	Centrally acting antiadrenergic agent
Therapeutic classification	Antihypertensive
Adverse reactions	
Central nervous system	Sedation, headache, asthenia, weakness, dizziness, decreased mental acuity, involuntary choreoathetoid movements, psychic disturbances, depression, nightmares
Gastrointestinal system	Dry mouth

Methylphenidate

Brand names	Ritalin, Ritalin SR
Pharmacologic classification	Piperidine central nervous system stimulant
Therapeutic classification	Central nervous system stimulant
Adverse reactions	
Central nervous system	Nervousness, insomnia, dizziness, headache,

akathisia, dyskinesia,
Gilles de la Tourette's
syndrome, seizures

Eyes, ears, nose, and throat   Dry throat
Gastrointestinal system   Anorexia

Metolazone

Brand name   Diulo, Mykrox, Zaroxolyn
Pharmacologic classification   Quinazoline derivative
                               (thiazide-like) diuretic
Therapeutic classification   Diuretic, antihypertensive
Adverse reactions
   Central nervous system   Dizziness, headache, fatigue
   Gastrointestinal system   Anorexia

Metoprolol

Brand name   Toprol XL, Lopressor
Pharmacologic classification   Beta-adrenergic blocking
                               agent
Therapeutic classification   Antihypertensive, adjunc-
                               tive treatment of acute
                               myocardial infarction
Adverse reactions
   Central nervous system   Fatigue, lethargy, dizziness

Molindone

Brand name   Moban

Pharmacologic classification	Dihydroindolone
Therapeutic classification	Antipsychotic
Adverse reactions	
Central nervous system	Extrapyramidal reactions, sedation, tardive dyskinesia, pseudoparkinsonism, EEG changes, dizziness
Eyes, ears, nose, and throat	Blurred vision
Gastrointestinal system	Dry mouth

Nadolol

Brand name	Corgard
Pharmacologic classification	Beta-adrenergic blocking agent
Therapeutic classification	Antihypertensive, antianginal
Adverse reactions	
Central nervous system	Lethargy, fatigue

Neostigmine

Brand names	Prostigmin
Pharmacologic classification	Cholinesterase inhibitor
Therapeutic classification	Muscle stimulant

Adverse reactions

Central nervous system	Dizziness, headache, muscle weakness, mental confusion, jitters
Eyes, ears, nose, and throat	Blurred vision
Gastrointestinal system	Excessive salivation

Nicardipine

Brand name	Cardene, Cardene IV, Cardene SR
Pharmacologic classification	Calcium channel blocker
Therapeutic classification	Antianginal, antihypertensive

Adverse reactions

| Central nervous system | Headache, dizziness, light-headedness, paresthesia, drowsiness, asthenia |
| Gastrointestinal system | Dry mouth |

Nifedipine

Brand name	Adalat, Adalat CC, Procardia, Procardia XL
Pharmacologic classification	Calcium channel blocker
Therapeutic classification	Antianginal

Adverse reactions

| Central nervous system | Dizziness, light-headedness, flushing, headache, weakness, syncope |

Nitroglycerin (glyceryl trinitrate)

Brand name	Deponit, Minitran, Nitro-Bid, Nitro-Bid IV, Nitrocine, Nitrodisc, Nitro-Dur, Nitrogard, Nitroglyn, Nitroject, Nitrol, Nitrolingual, Nitrong, Nitrostat, Trans-derm-Nitro, Tridil
Pharmacologic classification	Nitrate
Therapeutic classification	Antianginal, vasodilator
Adverse reactions	
Central nervous system	Dizziness, headache, weakness

Norepinephrine

Brand name	Levophed
Pharmacologic classification	Adrenergic (direct-acting)
Therapeutic classification	Vasopressor
Adverse reactions	
Central nervous system	Dizziness, headache, weakness, restlessness, anxiety, insomnia, tremor
Respiratory system	Respiratory difficulties

Nortriptyline

Brand name	Aventyl, Pamelor

Pharmacologic classification	Tricyclic antidepressant
Therapeutic classification	Antidepressant
Adverse reactions	
Central nervous system	Drowsiness, dizziness, excitation, tremors, weakness, headache, nervousness, seizures, extrapyramidal symptoms, EEG changes, confusion
Eyes, ears, nose, and throat	Blurred vision, tinnitus
Gastrointestinal system	Dry mouth, anorexia

Oxazepam

Brand name	Serax
Pharmacologic classification	Benzodiazepine
Therapeutic classification	Antianxiety agent, sedative-hypnotic
Adverse reactions	
Central nervous system	Drowsiness, lethargy, hangover, fainting

Papaverine

| Brand name | Cerespan, Genabid, Pavabid, Pavabid HP Capsulets, Pavabid Plateau Caps, Pavacels, Pavagen, Pavarine Span- |

	caps, Pavased, Pavatym, Paverolan Lanacaps
Pharmacologic classification	Benzylisoquinoline derivative
Therapeutic classification	Peripheral vasodilators
Adverse reactions	
Central nervous system	Headache, depression
Gastrointestinal system	Dry mouth
Respiratory system	Apnea

Paroxetine

Brand name	Paxil
Pharmacologic classification	Selective serotonin reuptake inhibitor
Therapeutic classification	Antidepressant
Adverse reactions	
Central nervous system	Somnolence, dizziness, insomnia, tremor, nervousness, anxiety, paresthesia, confusion
Eyes, ears, nose, and throat	Blurred vision, lump or tightness in throat
Gastrointestinal system	Dry mouth

Penbutolol

Brand name	Levatol
Pharmacologic classification	Beta-adrenergic blocking agent

Therapeutic classification	Antihypertensive
Adverse reactions	
Central nervous system	Syncope, dizziness, vertigo, headache, fatigue, paresthesia, hypoesthesia, hyperesthesia, lethargy, anxiety, nervousness, diminished concentration, sleep disturbances, nightmares, bizarre or frequent dreams, sedation, changes in behavior, reversible mental depression, catatonia, hallucinations, alterations of time perception, memory loss, emotional lability, lightheadedness
Gastrointestinal system	Dry mouth, taste alteration
Respiratory system	Respiratory distress, shortness of breath

Pentaerythritol

Brand name	Dilar, Duotrate, Naptrate, Pentritol, Pentylan, Peritrate, Peritrate SA, PETN
Pharmacologic classification	Nitrate

Therapeutic classification	Antianginal agent, vaso-dilator
Adverse reactions	
Central nervous system	Dizziness, headache, weakness

Pentobarbital

Brand name	Nembutal Sodium
Pharmacologic classification	Barbiturate
Therapeutic classification	Anticonvulsant, sedative-hypnotic
Adverse reactions	
Central nervous system	Drowsiness, lethargy, hangover, paradoxic excitement in elderly patients

Pergolide

Brand names	Permax
Pharmacologic classification	Ergot derivative
Therapeutic classification	Antiparkinsonian agent
Adverse reactions	
Central nervous system	Headache, asthenia, dyskinesia, dizziness, hallucinations, dystonia, confusion, somnolence, insomnia, anxiety, depression, tremor, abnormal dreams, personality dis-

order, psychosis, abnormal gait, akathisia, extrapyramidal syndrome, incoordination, akinesia, hypertonia, neuralgia, twitching

Eyes, ears, nose, and throat — Abnormal vision, diplopia
Gastrointestinal system — Dry mouth, anorexia

Perphenazine

Brand name	Trilafon, Trilafon Concentrate
Pharmacologic classification	Phenothiazine (piperazine derivative)
Therapeutic classification	Antipsychotic, antiemetic
Adverse reactions	
Central nervous system	Extrapyramidal reactions, tardive dyskinesia, sedation, pseudoparkinsonism, EEG changes, dizziness
Eyes, ears, nose, and throat	Blurred vision
Gastrointestinal system	Dry mouth

Phenacemide

Brand names	Phenurone
Pharmacologic classification	Substituted acetylurea derivative, open-chain hydantoin

Therapeutic classification	Anticonvulsant
Adverse reactions	
Central nervous system	Drowsiness, dizziness, insomnia, headache, paresthesia, depression, suicidal tendencies, aggressiveness
Gastrointestinal system	Anorexia

Phenelzine

Brand name	Nardil
Pharmacologic classification	Monoamine oxidase inhibitor
Therapeutic classification	Antidepressant
Adverse reactions	
Central nervous system	Dizziness, vertigo, headache, hyperactivity, hyperreflexia, tremors, muscle twitching, mania, jitters, insomnia, confusion, memory impairments, drowsiness, weakness, fatigue
Gastrointestinal system	Dry mouth, anorexia, nausea

Phenobarbital

Brand name	Barbita, Solfoton, Luminal Sodium

| Pharmacologic classification | Barbiturate |
| Therapeutic classification | Anticonvulsant, sedative hypnotic |

Adverse reactions
   Central nervous system   Drowsiness, lethargy, hangover, paradoxic excitement in elderly patients

Phenytoin

Brand name   Dilantin, Dilantin-30 Pediatric, Dilantin-125, Dilantin Infatabs, Phenytex

Pharmacologic classification   Hydantoin derivative

Therapeutic classification   Anticonvulsant

Adverse reactions
   Central nervous system   Ataxia, slurred speech, confusion, dizziness, insomnia, nervousness, twitching, headache

   Eyes, ears, nose, and throat   Nystagmus, diplopia, blurred vision

Pimozide

Brand name   Orap

Pharmacologic classification   Diphenylbutylpiperidine

Therapeutic classification   Antipsychotic

Adverse reactions

Central nervous system	Parkinsonian-like symptoms, dystonia, akathisia, hyper-reflexia, opisthotonos, oculogyric crisis, tardive dyskinesia, sedation
Eyes, ears, nose, and throat	Vision disturbances
Gastrointestinal system	Dry mouth

Pindolol

Brand name	Visken
Pharmacologic classification	Beta-adrenergic blocking agent
Therapeutic classification	Antihypertensive

Adverse reactions

Central nervous system	Insomnia, fatigue, dizziness, nervousness, vivid dreams, hallucinations, lethargy
Eyes, ears, nose, and throat	Vision disturbances

Piroxicam

Brand name	Feldene
Pharmacologic classification	Nonsteroidal anti-inflammatory
Therapeutic classification	Non-narcotic analgesic, antipyretic, anti-inflammatory

Adverse reactions
    Central nervous system   Headache, drowsiness, dizziness, paresthesia, somnolence
    Eyes, ears, nose, and throat   Auditory disturbances

Prazepam

Brand name   Centrax
Pharmacologic classification   Benzodiazepine
Therapeutic classification   Antianxiety agent
Adverse reactions
    Central nervous system   Drowsiness, lethargy, hangover, ataxia, dizziness, fainting
    Gastrointestinal system   Dry mouth

Prazosin

Brand name   Minipress
Pharmacologic classification   Alpha-antiadrenergic blocking agent
Therapeutic classification   Antihypertensive
Adverse reactions
    Central nervous system   Headache, weakness, dizziness, depression, drowsiness, first-dose syncope
    Eyes, ears, nose, and throat   Blurred vision
    Gastrointestinal system   Dry mouth

Prednisone

Brand name	Deltasone, Liquid Pred, Meticorten, Orasone, Panasol, Prednicen-M, Prednisone Intensol, Sterapred
Pharmacologic classification	Adrenocorticoid
Therapeutic classification	Anti-inflammatory, immunosuppressant
Adverse reactions	
Central nervous system	Euphoria, insomnia, psychotic behavior, pseudotumor cerebri

Primidone

Brand name	Mysoline
Pharmacologic classification	Barbiturate analogue
Therapeutic classification	Anticonvulsant
Adverse reactions	
Central nervous system	Drowsiness, ataxia, emotional disturbances, vertigo, hyperirritability, fatigue
Eyes, ears, nose, and throat	Diplopia, nystagmus
Gastrointestinal system	Anorexia

Prochlorperazine

Brand name	Compazine, Stemetil, Chlorpazine, Compazine Spansule, Compa-Z, Compazine Syrup, Cotranzine, Ultrazine-10
Pharmacologic classification	Phenothiazine
Therapeutic classification	Antipsychotic
Adverse reactions	
Central nervous system	Extrapyramidal reactions, sedation, pseudoparkinsonism, EEG changes, dizziness
Eyes, ears, nose, and throat	Blurred vision
Gastrointestinal system	Dry mouth

Procyclidine

Brand names	Kemadrin
Pharmacologic classification	Anticholinergic
Therapeutic classification	Antiparkinsonian agent
Adverse reactions	
Central nervous system	Light-headedness, giddiness
Eyes, ears, nose, and throat	Blurred vision
Gastrointestinal system	Dry mouth

Promazine

Brand name	Primazine, Prozine-50, Sparine
Pharmacologic classification	Aliphatic phenothiazine
Therapeutic classification	Antipsychotic
Adverse reactions	
Central nervous system	Extrapyramidal reactions, tardive dyskinesia, sedation, pseudoparkinsonism, EEG changes, dizziness
Eyes, ears, nose, and throat	Blurred vision
Gastrointestinal system	Dry mouth

Propranolol

Brand name	Inderal, Inderal LA
Pharmacologic classification	Beta-adrenergic blocking agent
Therapeutic classification	Antihypertensive, antianginal, antiarrhythmic, adjunctive treatment of acute myocardial infarction
Adverse reactions	
Central nervous system	Fatigue, lethargy, vivid dreams, hallucinations, mental depression

Protriptyline

Brand name	Vivactil
Pharmacologic classification	Tricyclic antidepressant
Therapeutic classification	Antidepressant
Adverse reactions	
Central nervous system	Excitation, tremors, weakness, headache, nervousness, seizures, EEG changes, extrapyramidal reactions, confusion
Eyes, ears, nose, and throat	Blurred vision, tinnitus
Gastrointestinal system	Dry mouth, anorexia

Pyridostigmine

Brand names	Mestinon, Mestinon Timespan, Regonol
Pharmacologic classification	Cholinesterase inhibitor
Therapeutic classification	Muscle stimulant
Adverse reactions	
Central nervous system	Headache (with high doses), weakness, seizures
Gastrointestinal system	Excessive salivation

Quazepam

Brand name	Doral
Pharmacologic classification	Benzodiazepine

Therapeutic classification	Hypnotic
Adverse reactions	
Central nervous system	Fatigue, dizziness, daytime drowsiness, headache

Quinapril

Brand name	Accupril
Pharmacologic classification	ACE inhibitor
Therapeutic classification	Antihypertensive
Adverse reactions	
Central nervous system	Somnolence, vertigo, light-headedness, syncope, nervousness, depression
Eyes, ears, nose, and throat	Cough, dry mouth or throat

Ramipril

Brand name	Altace
Pharmacologic classification	ACE inhibitor
Therapeutic classification	Antihypertensive
Adverse reactions	
Central nervous system	Headache, dizziness, fatigue, asthenia, malaise, light-headedness, anxiety, amnesia, seizures, depression, insomnia, nervousness, neuralgia, neuropathy, paresthesia, somnolence, tremor, vertigo

Eyes, ears, nose, and throat	Dysphagia, increased salivation
Gastrointestinal system	Anorexia, dry mouth, taste disturbance
Respiratory system	Dry, persistent, nonproductive cough

Reserpine

Brand name	Serpalan, Serpasil
Pharmacologic classification	Rauwolfia alkaloid, peripherally acting antiadrenergic agent
Therapeutic classification	Antihypertensive, antipsychotic
Adverse reactions	
Central nervous system	Mental confusion, depression, drowsiness, nervousness, paradoxic anxiety, nightmares, extrapyramidal symptoms, sedation
Gastrointestinal system	Dry mouth

Secobarbital

Brand name	Seconal Sodium
Pharmacologic classification	Barbiturate
Therapeutic classification	Anticonvulsant, sedative-hypnotic

Adverse reactions
    Central nervous system   Drowsiness, lethargy, hangover, paradoxic excitement in elderly patients

Selegiline

Brand name	Eldepryl
Pharmacologic classification	Monoamine oxidase inhibitor
Therapeutic classification	Antiparkinsonian agent

Adverse reactions
    Central nervous system   Dizziness, increased tremor, chorea, loss of balance, restlessness, increased bradykinesia, facial grimacing, stiff neck, dyskinesia, involuntary movements, twitching, increased apraxia, behavioral changes, fatigue, headache
    Gastrointestinal system   Dry mouth, dysphagia, anorexia

Sertraline

Brand name	Zoloft
Pharmacologic classification	Serotonin uptake inhibitor
Therapeutic classification	Antidepressant

Adverse reactions

Central nervous system	Headache, tremor, dizziness, insomnia, somnolence, syncope, paresthesia, hypoesthesia, hyperesthesia, twitching, hypertonia, confusion, ataxia, abnormal coordination or gait, vertigo, hyperkinesia, hypokinesia, mania
Eyes, ears, nose, and throat	Nystagmus
Gastrointestinal system	Dry mouth, anorexia, dysphagia

Sotalol

Brand name	Betapace
Pharmacologic classification	Beta-adrenergic blocking agent
Therapeutic classification	Antiarrhythmic

Adverse reactions

Central nervous system	Asthenia, headache, dizziness, weakness, fatigue

Sulfadiazine

Brand name	Microsulfon
Pharmacologic classification	Sulfonamide
Therapeutic classification	Antibiotic

Adverse reactions

Central nervous system	Headache, mental depression, convulsions, hallucinations
Gastrointestinal system	Nausea, vomiting, anorexia

Sulfamethoxazole

Brand name	Gantanol, Gantanol DS
Pharmacologic classification	Sulfonamide
Therapeutic classification	Antibiotic
Adverse reactions	
Central nervous system	Headache, mental depression, seizures, hallucinations
Gastrointestinal system	Nausea, vomiting, anorexia

Sulindac

Brand name	Clinoril
Pharmacologic classification	Nonsteroidal anti-inflammatory
Therapeutic classification	Non-narcotic analgesic, antipyretic, anti-inflammatory
Adverse reactions	
Central nervous system	Headache, dizziness, nervousness, delirium, psychosis, neuropathy, hallucinations, aseptic meningitis

Eyes, ears, nose, and throat   Transient visual distur-
                                bances, tinnitus

Tacrine

Brand name   Cognex
Pharmacologic classification   Centrally acting reversible
                                cholinesterase inhibitor
Therapeutic classification   Psychotherapeutic agent
                                (for Alzheimer's disease)
Adverse reactions
  Central nervous system   Agitation, ataxia
  Gastrointestinal system   Anorexia, nausea, vomiting

Temazepam

Brand name   Restoril
Pharmacologic classification   Benzodiazepine
Therapeutic classification   Sedative-hypnotic
Adverse reactions
  Central nervous system   Confusion, dizziness,
                                drowsiness, lethargy, dis-
                                turbed coordination, day-
                                time sedation
  Gastrointestinal system   Anorexia

Terazosin

Brand name   Hytrin
Pharmacologic classification   Selective alpha blocker

Therapeutic classification	Antihypertensive
Adverse reactions	
Central nervous system	Asthenia, dizziness, headache, nervousness, paresthesia, somnolence
Eyes, ears, nose, and throat	Blurred vision

Terbutaline

Brand name	Brethaire, Brethine, Bricanyl
Pharmacologic classification	Adrenergic
Therapeutic classification	Bronchodilator, premature labor inhibitor
Adverse reactions	
Central nervous system	Nervousness, tremors, headache, drowsiness

Thioridazine

Brand name	Mellaril, Mellaril Concentrate
Pharmacologic classification	Phenothiazine
Therapeutic classification	Antipsychotic
Adverse reactions	
Central nervous system	Extrapyramidal reactions, tardive dyskinesia, sedation, EEG changes, dizziness
Eyes, ears, nose, and throat	Blurred vision

Gastrointestinal system   Dry mouth

Timolol

Brand name   Blocadren
Pharmacologic classification   Beta-adrenergic blocking
                                    agent
Therapeutic classification   Antihypertensive agent,
                                    adjunct in myocardial
                                    infarction, anti-glaucoma
                                    agent

Adverse reactions
  Central nervous system   Fatigue, lethargy, vivid
                                    dreams

Tobramycin

Brand names   Nebcin
Pharmacologic classification   Aminoglycoside
Therapeutic classification   Antibiotic
Adverse reactions
  Central nervous system   Headache, lethargy, neuro-
                                    muscular blockade
  Eyes, ears, nose, and throat   Ototoxicity (i.e., tinnitus,
                                    vertigo, hearing loss)

Tolmetin

Brand name   Tolectin-200, Tolectin-400,
                                    Tolectin-600, Tolectin DS

Pharmacologic classification	Nonsteroidal anti-inflammatory
Therapeutic classification	Non-narcotic analgesic, antipyretic, anti-inflammatory
Adverse reactions	
Central nervous system	Headache, drowsiness, dizziness
Eyes, ears, nose, and throat	Tinnitus, visual disturbances

Tranylcypromine

Brand name	Parnate
Pharmacologic classification	Monoamine oxidase inhibitor
Therapeutic classification	Antidepressant
Adverse reactions	
Central nervous system	Dizziness, vertigo, headache, overstimulation, numbness, paresthesia, tremors, jitters, confusion, memory impairment
Eyes, ears, nose, and throat	Blurred vision, tinnitus
Gastrointestinal system	Dry mouth, anorexia, nausea

Trazodone

Brand name	Desyrel, Trazon, Trialodine

Pharmacologic classification	Triazolopyridine derivative
Therapeutic classification	Antidepressant
Adverse reactions	
Central nervous system	Drowsiness, dizziness, tremors, weakness, nervousness, fatigue, confusion, vivid dreams and nightmares, anger, hostility
Eyes, ears, nose, and throat	Blurred vision, tinnitus
Gastrointestinal system	Dry mouth, anorexia

Triamterene

Brand name	Dyrenium
Pharmacologic classification	Potassium-sparing diuretic
Therapeutic classification	Diuretic
Adverse reactions	
Central nervous system	Dizziness, weakness, fatigue, headache
Gastrointestinal system	Dry mouth

Triazolam

Brand name	Halcion
Pharmacologic classification	Benzodiazepine
Therapeutic classification	Sedative-hypnotic
Adverse reactions	
Central nervous system	Drowsiness, dizziness, headache, rebound

insomnia, light-headedness, lack of coordination, amnesia, mental confusion, depression,

Trifluoperazine

Brand name	Stelazine, Stelazine Concentrate
Pharmacologic classification	Piperazine phenothiazine
Therapeutic classification	Antipsychotic
Adverse reactions	
Central nervous system	Extrapyramidal reactions, tardive dyskinesia, pseudoparkinsonism, dizziness, drowsiness, insomnia
Eyes, ears, nose, and throat	Blurred vision
Gastrointestinal system	Dry mouth

Trihexyphenidyl

Brand name	Artane, Artane Sequels, Trihexane, Trihexy-2, Trihexy-5
Pharmacologic classification	Anticholinergic
Therapeutic classification	Antiparkinsonian agent
Adverse reactions	
Central nervous system	Nervousness, dizziness, headache, restlessness,

hallucinations, euphoria,
amnesia

Eyes, ears, nose, and throat	Blurred vision
Gastrointestinal system	Dry mouth

Trimipramine

Brand name	Surmontil
Pharmacologic classification	Tricyclic antidepressant
Therapeutic classification	Antidepressant, antianxiety agent

Adverse reactions
    Central nervous system   Drowsiness, dizziness, excitation, tremors, weakness, headache, nervousness, EEG changes, seizures, extrapyramidal reactions, confusion

Eyes, ears, nose, and throat	Blurred vision, tinnitus
Gastrointestinal system	Dry mouth, anorexia

Valproate

Valproic acid

Divalproex

Brand names	Depakene Syrup, Myproic Acid Syrup (brand names for valproate)

	Depakene, Myproic Acid (brand names for valproic acid)
	Depakote, Depakote Sprinkle (brand names for divalproex)
Pharmacologic classification	Carboxylic acid derivative
Therapeutic classification	Anticonvulsant
Adverse reactions	
Central nervous system	Sedation, emotional upset, depression, psychosis, aggressiveness, hyperactivity, behavioral deterioration, muscle weakness, tremors
Gastrointestinal system	Anorexia

Verapamil

Brand name	Calan, Calan SR, Isoptin, Isoptin SR, Verelan
Pharmacologic classification	Calcium channel blocker
Therapeutic classification	Antianginal, antihypertensive, antiarrhythmic
Adverse reactions	
Central nervous system	Dizziness, headache, fatigue

Glossary

VENTILATOR TERMINOLOGY

Abscess — Localized collection of pus in a cavity formed by tissue degeneration

Acidosis — A condition of either respiratory or metabolic origin in which there are excessive quantities of acids in the blood

Acute respiratory failure — A sudden, life-threatening condition characterized by difficulty in breathing, excessively low levels of oxygen, and excessively high levels of carbon dioxide in the blood

Adult respiratory distress syndrome — A form of pulmonary edema resulting from marked, widespread damage to the alveolar-capillary membrane

Air-trapping — Abnormal condition in which air cannot be expelled from the alveoli during exhalation as a result of collapse of the bronchioles or blockage by tenacious mucus

Alkalosis — A condition, of either respiratory or metabolic origin, in which there is an excessive alkaline content in the blood

Alveoli — Microscopic air sacs located at the end of the respiratory tract where gas exchange with the blood takes place

Anoxia — Without oxygen

Apnea — Absence of breathing; apnea during the respiratory cycle usually results from a lack of stimulation to the respiratory center, secondary to inadequate carbon dioxide levels in the blood

Assist control (A/C) — A mode of mechanical ventilatory support in which the ventilator responds to the patient's spontaneous breathing efforts by delivering volume and providing a preset number of breaths if the patient fails to inspire within a set time period

Atelectasis — An area of collapsed lung that occurs when all of the oxygen in the tissue is absorbed by the blood and access to further oxygenation through the bronchioles is blocked; may occur if the bronchioles are blocked with secretions

Atrophy — Wasting away of tissues, organs, or the entire body as from disease or death and reabsorption of cells

Auscultate — To listen (e.g., as to chest sounds with a stethoscope)

Bilevel ventilation — A variation of continuous positive airway pressure; a method of noninvasive mechanical ventilation that provides an inspiratory pressure as well as a lower expiratory pressure

Blebs — A blister or bubble in the lungs; in emphysema, a bleb is a large area in which the alveolar walls have deteriorated, forming an air sac; blebs are sometimes large enough to contain several milliliters of trapped air or liquid secretions

Bronchi — The air passages of the lungs, beginning with the first bifurcation through all their branches to the smallest tubes at the distal portions of the lungs

Bronchiectasis — Chronic dilation of the bronchi and bronchioles with secondary infection and destruction of lung tissue; characterized by secretions with a pungent odor

Bronchiole — The smallest conducting airway with cartilage construction in the respiratory tract; the bronchioles connect to the alveoli to complete the lung unit

Bronchodilators — Any of a number of drugs that will enlarge the bronchial air passage either by shrinking the mucous membranes or by relaxing the smooth muscles that constrict the air passages

Bronchorrhea — An abnormal condition in which the bronchial mucous membranes secrete an excessive amount of mucus

Bronchoscopy — A method of viewing inside the trachea and main bronchial tubes by means of a tube and light that are passed through the mouth into the trachea and bronchi

Cheyne-Stokes respiration — Abnormal respiration that is intermittently deep and shallow and then ceases temporarily before beginning again; the apnea may last from 10 seconds to 1 minute

Chronic obstructive pulmonary disease (COPD) — A disease that is characterized by generalized airway obstruction; a combination of emphysema and bronchitis, sometimes with components of asthma

Congestive heart failure (CHF) — A chronic failure of the heart to pump adequate amounts of blood throughout the body; results in congestion and fluid accumulate in various organs in the body.

Continuous positive airway pressure (CPAP) — A mode of mechanical ventilatory support that is noncycled, maintains positive pressure in the airways throughout the respiratory cycle, and increases oxygenation by enhancing functional residual capacity (FRC) and lung compliance; used for patients who are breathing spontaneously but who have inadequate oxygenation because of decreased FRC, for patients who are weaning from mechanical ventilation, and to treat patients with sleep apnea. CPAP allows the patient to exhale against the positive pressure. The continuous positive pressure is applied with an endotracheal, nasotracheal, or tracheostomy tube or through a continuous-flow, tight-fitting face mask.

Controlled mode ventilation (CMV) — A mode of ventilation that cycles to provide inspiratory breaths independent of the patient's breathing efforts

Cor pulmonale — Heart disease that occurs after lung disease and strains the right ventricle; chronic cor pulmonale is characterized by hypertrophy of the right ventricle resulting from lung disease; acute cor pulmonale is characterized by dilation and failure of the right side of the heart due to pulmonary embolism

Coryza — Common cold

Costal breathing — Respiration produced solely by use of the intercostal muscles

Cuff — The balloon-like part of an artificial airway that is inflated in the trachea to provide a seal in the airway

Cyanosis — A bluish discoloration of the skin and mucous membrane indicating inadequate oxygenation

Dead space, anatomic — The air that is always in the tube system of the lungs, normally 150 ml in the normal adult or approximately 1 ml/lb of body weight

Decannulation — The removal of a tracheotomy tube

Dyspnea — Labored breathing; shortness of breath

Embolism — Obstruction of a vessel by an embolus

Embolus — A globule of fat, a clot, or a gas bubble circulating in the bloodstream that obstructs the blood flow

Emesis — The act of vomiting

Emphysema — Air trapped in the lungs or tissue as a result of a disease process, aging, or both

Exhaled tidal volume — The amount of volume that a patient receiving mechanical ventilation exhales or returns to the ventilator

Expectoration — The act of coughing up and spitting out material (i.e., sputum) from the lungs and trachea

Extubation — The removal of an endotracheal tube

Exudate — Any fluid exuded out of a tissue or its capillaries, more specifically because of injury or inflammation; contains microorganisms and cells

Fenestration — An opening or window; a fenestrated tracheostomy tube aids the passage of air through the cannula

Fistula — An abnormal opening or hole from a hollow organ to the surface or from one organ to another; formed by incomplete closure of a wound or abscess, such as a tracheoesophageal fistula

Guillain-Barré syndrome — Diffuse infection or irritation of nerves that can affect the respiratory system by causing paralysis of the muscles for breathing; a type of polyneuritis

Hemoptysis — Spitting or coughing blood or blood-tinged mucus

Hypercapnia — The presence of excessively high levels of arterial carbon dioxide

Hypocapnia — Abnormally decreased arterial carbon dioxide; alkalosis

Hypoxemia — Insufficient amounts of oxygenation in the arterial blood

Hypoxia — Inadequate tissue oxygenation

Inner cannula — The internal portion of a tracheostomy tube that fits within the main or external structure of the tube

Intermittent mandatory ventilation (IMV) — A mode of cycled ventilation in which the patient may breathe spontaneously between timed mandatory breaths

Intermittent positive pressure ventilation (IPPV) — A mode of ventilation in which the ventilator provides positive pressure and inflates the lungs; also referred to as inspiratory positive pressure breathing

Intubation — Insertion of an endotracheal tube through the nose or mouth into the trachea

Ischemia — A decrease in blood supply to a localized area as a result of constriction of blood vessels

Laryngitis — Inflammation of the larynx that may obstruct ventilation

Lobectomy — Removal of a lobe of a lung

Lung abscess — Enclosed pus-filled area or cavity inside the lung

Maximum ventilatory volume — The maximum volume of air a patient can move in a minute; previously called maximum breathing capacity

Mediastinum — The area inside the thoracic cavity directly behind the sternum and between the two lungs; contains the heart, trachea, esophagus, large blood vessels, and nerves

Minimal leak technique — The process of maintaining cuff inflation with a small air leak to ensure that the cuff does not place excessive pressure on the tracheal walls

Mucolytic — A pharmacologic agent used to loosen mucus for easier removal from the airway

Mucus plug — Thick, dry pieces of mucus that are of a size to occlude the lumen of a bronchi or bronchiole

Myasthenia gravis — A chronic progressive muscular weakness beginning usually in the face and throat

Negative pressure ventilation — A noninvasive mode of ventilatory support that makes use of negative pressure around the thorax to decrease intrathoracic pressure in relation to atmospheric pressure, causing inspiration; expiration is passive

One-way (speaking) valve — A one-way valve that is placed on the hub of a tracheostomy tube to allow air to enter on inspiration; on expiration the valve closes, and the air is redirected through the vocal folds and into the upper airway, allowing the patient to speak and swallow

Orthopnea — Discomfort in breathing except when sitting or upright

Oxyhemoglobin — The combination of oxygen and hemoglobin

Outer cannula — The portion of the tracheostomy tube that forms the actual body of the tube; the external structure of the tube into which the inner cannula fits

Partial leak — A leak maintained in a tracheostomy tube cuff that allows a patient access to airflow through the upper airway for the purposes of speaking, swallowing, and airway clearance

Positive end expiratory pressure (PEEP) — A form of mechanical ventilation that applies positive pressure at the end of each expiration to keep open collapsed alveoli; used for a patient who is not breathing spontaneously and may be administered with positive-pressure mechanical ventilation; also may be performed during manual ventilation by attaching a PEEP valve to the manual resuscitation bag. It is used to treat patients with diffuse restrictive lung disease or hypoxemic respiratory failure that is unresponsive to mechanically delivered oxygen alone.

Pickwickian syndrome — A restrictive disease of the chest that is caused by obesity and characterized by somnolence, hypoventilation, and erythrocytosis

Pleura — The serous membrane enveloping the lungs and lining the walls of the pleural cavity

Positive pressure ventilation — A means of mechanical ventilation that can be administered via invasive or noninvasive means by creating a higher pressure than atmospheric to push air into the lungs

Pneumonia — Inflammation of the lung parenchyma characterized by consolidation of the affected part

Pneumonitis — Inflammation of the lungs; often a viral pneumonia

Pneumothorax — The presence of air or gas in the pleural cavity; will result in a collapsed lung if left uncorrected

Pulmonary bullae — Large blebs or blisters inside the lungs, as in emphysema

Pulmonary edema — Swelling of alveoli in the lungs that occurs when they fill with fluid leaking from the capillaries; can lead to significant respiratory distress

Pulmonary emboli — Blood clots in the vessels of the lungs; can be fatal

Pulse oximetry — A noninvasive method of determining arterial oxygen saturation using a probe placed on a highly oxygenated area of the body

Purulent — Containing, consisting of, or forming pus

Rales — Adventitious lung sounds arising from fluid in the lungs at an alveolar level that do not clear with a cough

Rhonchi — Adventitious lung sounds arising from fluid in the bronchi and bronchioles that clear with a cough.

Sigh — Deep breath normally taken about every 10 minutes

Spirometer — Instrument that measures vital capacity or volume of inhaled and exhaled air

Sputum — Coughed or expectorated secretions of the lungs, bronchi, and trachea

Stridor — Abnormal, harsh, high-pitched sounds that occur during difficult or obstructed respiration

Synchronized intermittent mandatory ventilation (SIMV) — A mode of cycled ventilation in which the patient can breathe spontaneously between timed breaths; unlike intermittent mandatory ventilation, this mode of ventilation will synchronize with the spontaneous breathing efforts of the patient and wait for a preset time to allow the patient to inspire before imposing a preset breath

Tachycardia — Increased heart rate, usually greater than 100 beats per minute

Tachypnea — Abnormally fast breathing

Talking tracheostomy tube — A tracheostomy tube that has been adapted to permit phonation in the presence of an inflated cuff; talking tracheostomy tubes contain an external air port that connects to a separate air source and allows air to enter the airway above the level of the tracheostomy tube cuff

Tidal volume — The amount of air passing in and out of the lungs during normal resting respiration

Tracheostomy — Formation of an opening into the trachea; the tube used to secure the stoma after a tracheotomy

Tracheotomy — The operation of opening into the trachea

Weaning — The process of removing a patient from mechanical ventilation

NEONATAL INTENSIVE CARE UNIT TERMINOLOGY

Adjusted chronologic age (ACA) — The age a preterm infant would be if he or she had been born at term; used in assessing developmental appropriateness of specific skills and milestones at a given point in time; agreed to be appropriate for assessing physical, cognitive, and language development up to 12 months' corrected age; some experts believe that age should be corrected up to 24 months to assess the child's development fairly

Anencephaly — Literally means without brain; refers to a child with a severely malformed, poorly developed brain

Aspirate — To breathe material into the trachea or lungs; to draw out such material by suction

Auditory brain stem evoked response testing (ABER) — A form of auditory evoked potential response testing in which the neurophysiologic behavior of the auditory mechanism is measured

Auditory evoked potential response — The neurophysiologic response of the auditory system to auditory stimulation, which is measured using electrophysiologic devices

Bronchopulmonary dysplasia (BPD) — Chronic pulmonary insufficiency arising from long-term artificial pulmonary ventilation; seen more frequently in premature infants than in mature infants

Bilirubin — Breakdown product of the blood which can cause jaundice

Bradycardia — A heart rate that is slower than normal

Chest tube — A tube placed in the chest cavity and connected to a suction system to remove trapped air or fluid, allowing the lungs to expand; used to treat pneumothorax

Cytomegalovirus (CMV) — A common virus that is detrimental and possibly lethal to the developing fetus; may cause birth defects and mental retardation

Endotracheal tube — A stiff plastic tube that is passed through the mouth into the trachea and connected to a respirator

Failure to thrive (FTT) — A condition diagnosed in the first 2 years of life in which a child's weight drops below the third percentile of growth with no known organic etiology

Full-term infant — Infant whose gestational age is between 38 and 42 weeks

Gavage feeding — A method of feeding breast milk or formula through a small tube passed through the baby's mouth or nose into the esophagus

Gestational age — Number of weeks the baby is carried in the mother's womb

Gravida — A term used to specify pregnancy; modification is usually by number (e.g., primigravida is the first pregnancy)

Haberman feeder — A specially designed infant feeder for use with cleft palate infants

Hyaline membrane disease — A respiratory disorder often seen in premature babies in which there is a tendency for the tiny air sacs of the lungs to collapse, usually due to underdevelopment

Hydrocephalus — An accumulation of cerebrospinal fluid in the head that can create increased pressure on the brain and cause permanent brain damage

Hyperbilirubinemia — Excessive supply of bilirubin, commonly referred to as jaundice; can cause liver damage and, in extreme cases, brain damage or death if untreated

Incubator — A special enclosed bed for infants in which the temperature may be controlled

Intrauterine growth retardation (IUGR) — Small, thin, malnourished infant; malnourishment is caused by a placental insufficiency of some sort; characterized by irritable, frequent crying

Intraventricular hemorrhage (IVH) — Hemorrhage occurring within a ventricle of the brain or heart; the extent of the bleeding is designated by assignment of a grade; grade I is least extensive; grade IV is most extensive

Jaundice — A yellowish staining of the skin, sclerae, and deeper tissues caused by too much bilirubin in the blood

Low birth weight (LBW) — Weight less than normal for an infant's gestational age due to various reasons including genetic, drug exposure, and maternal malnutrition

Meconium — A dark green material found in the newborn's intestine; the first stool an infant passes

Microcephaly — Literally means small head; may be associated with premature fusion of the bones of the skull of an infant;

can restrict brain growth and cause mental retardation if untreated

Möbius' syndrome — Congenital facial diplegia; a developmental bilateral facial paralysis usually associated with oculomotor or other neurologic disorders

Monitor — Machine used to observe and record such functions as breathing, temperature, and heart rate

Neonate — A newborn infant

Neonatologist — A physician whose medical specialty deals with the care of newborns

Open radiant warmer — An open bed with an overhead warmer that helps keep the baby warm; with this bed, several people can care for the baby at one time

Oxygen saturation monitor — A device that monitors the oxygen saturation in the blood; oxygen saturation is a measurement of the percentage of oxygen combined with hemoglobin relative to the maximum amount of oxygen the hemoglobin can contain

Oxyhood — A plastic box that fits over the baby's head to provide oxygen and moisture

Phenylketonuria (PKU) — A disorder of metabolism that allows accumulation of excessive phenylalanine in the brain tissues; can lead to mental retardation

Phototherapy — A method of treating jaundice by placing lights (Bililights) over the baby's bed to help break down bilirubin; the light causes the breakdown of bilirubin and excretion through urine and stool

Post-term delivery — Delivery of an infant after the thirty-ninth week of gestation

Premature infant — An infant who is born before 38 weeks of gestational age

Respirator — An apparatus for administering artificial respiration

Respiratory distress syndrome (RDS) — A set of symptoms resulting from oxygen deprivation in the perinatal period; often associated with bronchopulmonary dysplasia

Short-bowel syndrome (short-gut syndrome) — The state of malabsorption and subsequent malnutrition that is induced after a massive small intestinal resection; some causes include necrotizing enterocolitis, midgut volvulus, multiple intestinal atresias, intestinal malrotation, and abdominal wall defects

Surfactant — A substance used in the perinatal period to treat respiratory problems common to premature infants

Syndactyly — Webbing between the fingers or toes; a condition common to some syndromes that also involve anomalies of the head and neck

TORCH syndrome — Infection in newborns attributable to any combination of toxoplasmosis, rubella, cytomegalovirus, and herpes viruses; places the infant at risk for hearing loss and language problems

Index